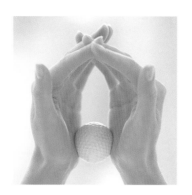

reflexology

health at your fingertips

D1350270

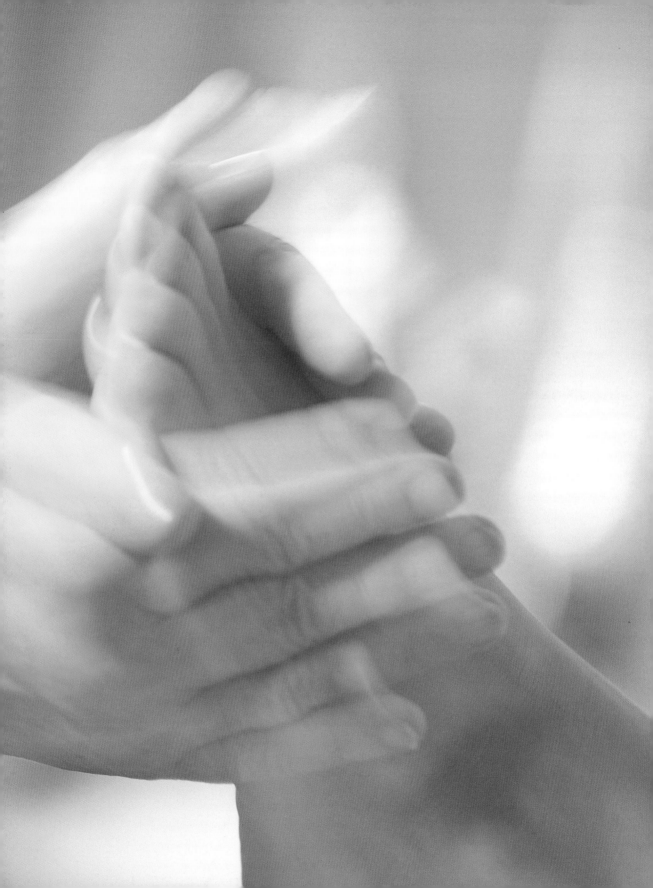

reflexology
health at your fingertips

BARBARA & KEVIN KUNZ

PHOTOGRAPHY BY RUTH JENKINSON

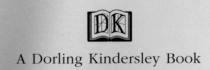

A Dorling Kindersley Book

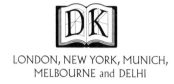

LONDON, NEW YORK, MUNICH,
MELBOURNE and DELHI

Editor: Shannon Beatty   **Designer:** Mark Cavanagh
Senior Editor: Penny Warren   **Senior Art Editor:** Margherita Gianni
Managing Editor: Stephanie Farrow   **Managing Art Editor:** Mabel Chan
DTP Designer: Sonia Charbonnier   **Category Publisher:** Mary-Clare Jerram
Art Director: Carole Ash   **Production Controller:** Louise Daly

First published in Great Britain in 2003
by Dorling Kindersley Limited,
80 Strand, London WC2R 0RL
A Penguin Company

8 10 9 7 6

A CIP catalogue record for this book is
available from the British Library.

ISBN 0 7513 6448 7

Colour reproduced by Colourscan, Singapore

Printed and bound in Singapore by Star Standard

See our complete catalogue at www.dk.com

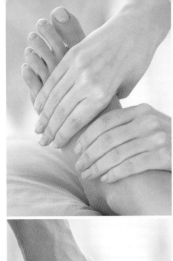

CONTENTS

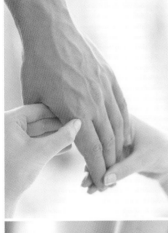

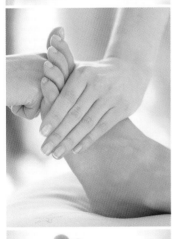

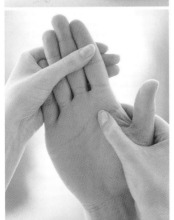

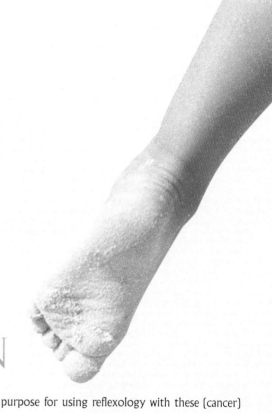

INTRODUCTION

After 27 years as professional reflexologists, authors and teachers, we can — and will in this book — tell you about reflexology's history and theory, its benefits and research, the techniques and the charts and the approaches to health concerns. In this introduction, however, we would like to tell you about why reflexology means so much to so many.

It has always struck us that the motivation to work with reflexology, for so many people, is a personal one. The desire to help other people is deeply embedded in the ethos and practice of reflexology. We once asked reflexologists why they had become reflexologists. The answer from practitioners in 11 different countries was 100 per cent unanimous — to help people.

As Barbara Dobbs observed in her ground-breaking study, "Alternative Health Approaches", published in *Nursing Mirror* (vol. 160, no. 9, February 27, 1985):

"Our purpose for using reflexology with these (cancer) patients was to decrease their pain but we soon realised the beneficial effect of reflexology on the morale of patients and families. Something was being done for them. Patients expressed feelings of being less abandoned and the families expressed satisfaction at seeing that something painless existed that could aid their relative. In three situations we taught a relative how to use reflexology and the benefit seemed to have been as important for the relative as for the patient…Patients' comments about reflexology seem to show that it could be one way for them to feel this support and to have a helping presence near them in their last days. The family member felt that a contribution was being made to a loved one's well-being. The patient experienced a tangible support from a loved one."

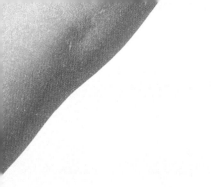
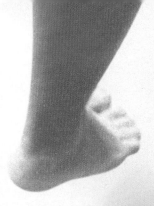

The mother of a child partially blinded through an accident helped introduce us to reflexology. After she had used reflexology to overcome her own arthritis, she then applied her skills to help her child's blinded eye track more normally. Another friend of ours had a daughter for whom the doctors recommended institutionalisation, as they did not expect her to recover sufficiently from a car accident to be able to live independently. Following her mother's reflexology work, however, the daughter returned to her teaching job.

In another similar instance, a retired schoolteacher initially took our reflexology class in order to improve the mobility of his arthritic hands. However, his ultimate goal was to enable himself to apply reflexology techniques to his wife. When we met his wife, it became clear why he was so interested in helping her — she had been impaired by a stroke, and he wanted to show that he cared, in addition to improving her condition.

Can reflexology help you to help a loved one? As you read this book and learn to apply reflexology techniques, you can see first-hand how it can help you improve your own health as well as that of a loved one. Keeping yourself healthy is beneficial to others. Like the retired schoolteacher, through applying reflexology work to someone else, you will receive the benefit of knowing you reached out to help.

Barbara K. Kunz

Kevin M. Kunz

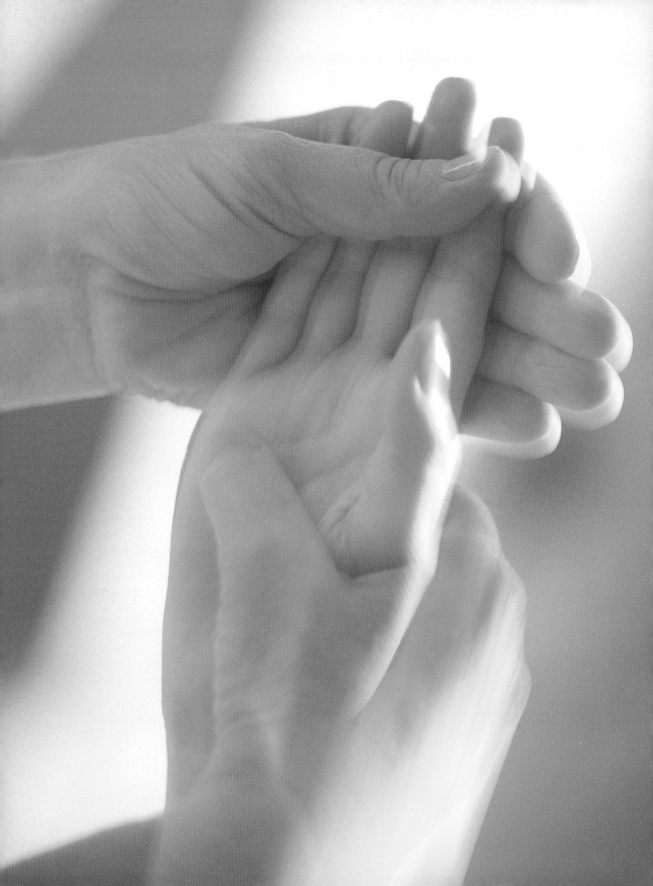

PRINCIPLES OF REFLEXOLOGY

Reflexology is the practice of applying pressure to specific points on the feet and hands to influence the health of corresponding parts of the body. "Pressure sensors" on the hands and feet connect with different parts of the body, and as reflexology techniques stimulate these sensors, waves of relaxation are sent throughout the body. In this section we outline the principles and history of reflexology, and reveal how it is used to aid health and encourage relaxation, prevent disease, reduce pain and improve quality of life.

THE HISTORY OF REFLEXOLOGY

Modern reflexology has its origins in the 19th century and became fully developed in the 1930s, when Eunice Ingham and others devised charts of reflex zones for the hands and feet. However, archaeological evidence suggests that applying pressure to hands and feet is an ancient tradition. There are Egyptian pictographs dating from 2330 BCE, for example, which depict work on the feet and hands.

Although the exact terminology and principles used remain unrecorded or have been lost during the course of history, archaeological artefacts demonstrate that the clear intent of some healers in ancient societies was to better health and prevent disease by applying pressure to the feet and hands.

ANCIENT EGYPT

Artefacts found in Egypt offer the clearest evidence of foot-work in ancient history. For example, at the entrance to the Tomb of the Physician Ankhmahor at Saqqara is a pictograph dating from 2330 BCE depicting work on the feet and hands. The prominent placement of such a pictograph on a tomb usually denotes

Artefacts show clearly that in ancient Egypt foot-work was considered a medical practice.

activities associated with the inhabitant's livelihood. One might infer that this person was a physician who practised foot-work. Intriguing to reflexologists is the translation of the hieroglyph, "Do not let it be painful" and "I do as you say" – similar interchanges still take place in reflexology practices today.

Another pictograph, found at the temple of Amon at Karnak, commemorating a military victory of Ramses II, who reigned 1279–13 BCE, shows a healer tending to the feet of foot soldiers at the battle of Qadesh. This military campaign of 1276 BCE involved a long march and, presumably, many foot-sore soldiers. Such pictographs make perfect sense to reflexologists, who often find themselves fighting the battle of tired feet on behalf of foot-sore clients. Historians record that Roman military leader Mark Antony (83–30 BCE) rubbed the feet of the Egyptian Queen Cleopatra VII (69–30 BCE) – Emperor Octavian (62–14 CE) writes of Antony's "pathetic enslavement...he even massaged her feet at dinner parties." To reflexologists, the image of Antony working on his lover's feet conjures an image of one person reaching out to another, bypassing words.

ANCIENT CHINA

Traditional Chinese Medicine (TCM) attributes good health to the free flow of *qi* energy through the body along energy channels, or meridians, which begin and extend down to the feet and hands, and can be manipulated to ensure a well-balanced flow through pressure on vital points. The Chinese first began using the concept of reflexology roughly 5,000 years ago. *The Method of Toe Observations*, recorded around that time in a Chinese medical text, the *Hwang Tee Internal Text*, attests to interest in the foot and its connection to

Some of the earliest evidence of foot-work comes from ancient Egypt, such as this relief (*right*) from the chapel of the Vizier Ptahhotep II at Saqqara, dated *c*. 2350 BCE.

general health. About 3,000 years later, a doctor in China devised the *Tao of Foot Centre*, a book that investigated and systemised the ancient teachings of *Examining Foot Method*.

After changes of dynasties, however, the Emperor of China's new Qin Dynasty ordered the burning of all books, perhaps including the *Tao of Foot Centre*, which may explain the decline in its teachings. Another possible explanation for its decline may be the rise in popularity of acupuncture. This tradition could be responsible for displacing that of foot-work, causing it to be largely forgotten in urban China. Luckily, rural villagers continued to practise this ancient precursor to modern reflexology, thereby keeping the tradition alive and primed for re-discovery in the 20th century.

JAPAN

The potent symbol of the foot in Japanese culture, spirituality and healing is revealed in the legendary footprint (697 CE) of Buddha etched on the upraised foot of the seated Buddha figure at the *Yakushiji* (Medicine Teacher's) Temple at Nara, Japan. Also in the temple grounds is found the *Bussokudo*, a building housing the famous stone footprint of Buddha, the *Bus–soku–seki*. Signifying the contact of Buddha with the earth, such footprints have lost their exact meanings, but their very existence illustrates the symbolic importance of feet in Buddhism and the diverse cultures of the East: similar footprints dating from the 4th century BCE exist in 15 other countries, including India, China, Thailand and Malaysia.

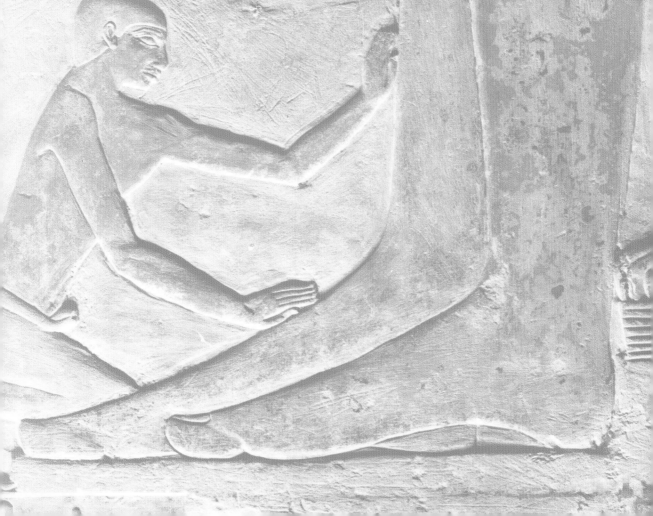

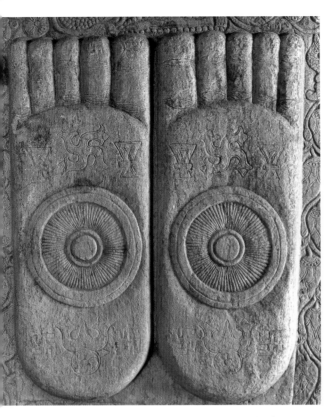

This 1st-century BCE Indian carving of Buddha's "foot-prints" symbolises the "grounding of the transcendent." The feet have long been a focus of respect in India.

OTHER CULTURES

Beliefs of many ancient cultures in diverse parts of the globe illustrate the special role of the foot in their societies. As Barbara Walker writes in *The Woman's Dictionary of Symbols and Other Sacred Objects* (1988), "Egyptians, Babylonians and other ancient people considered it essential to step on sacred ground with bare feet to absorb the holy influences from Mother Earth." Even now, the Kogi tribal people who live in Colombia in South America have a similar ancient belief. They consider that footwear cuts off their contact with Mother Earth. As a result, the Kogi today still go barefoot. In addition in Russia, the idea of walking barefoot on natural surfaces to benefit the body prevails, while many societies in Asia, Africa,

Germany and India have customs that involve work on the feet for health purposes. These examples suggest that many traditional societies see the foot as a conduit to spirituality and general wellness.

WESTERN IDEAS

The concept of reflexology as a medical therapy began to emerge in the 19th century, based on research by Western scientists and medical practitioners into the nervous system. Their basic discovery – that one can influence health and well-being through reflex actions – established the basis of all reflexologists' practice today.

The nervous system detects and interprets information from the outside world, and initialises the body's response to it. As part of their work, medical researchers in the 1800s studied the concept of the reflex and determined that it was "an involuntary response to a stimulus." They then began to explore the idea of "reflexes" and their effect on the body's state of health. Heat, cold, plasters and herbal poultices were applied to one part of the body – the reflex area – with the aim of influencing another part of the body. For example, a poultice applied to the surface of the skin on the chest was shown to influence the lungs beneath. The concept of "zones of influence" – in which an action performed on one part of the body causes a reaction in another part of the body – sought to explain such phenomena. As one of the many medical articles of the time expounded, "Reflex Action (is seen) as a Cause of Disease and (a) Means of Cure".

BRITISH DEVELOPMENTS

In 1893, Sir Henry Head (1861–1940) made a breakthrough in the understanding of the nervous system. He discovered that areas of hyperalgesia on the surface of the body (skin that is abnormally sensitive to pain) could occur as a result of a diseased internal organ. The connection, he found, was that the organ and area of skin were served by nerves emanating from the same segment of the spinal cord. His model showing how the skin and parts of the body are linked became known as "Head's Zones"; areas of skin linked by the nervous system to other parts of the body are now called "dermatomes". Doctors were able to refine their knowledge of this model in World War I (1914–18), observing that bullet wounds could cause pain not only in the damaged part of the body but all along the relevant nerve pathway.

RUSSIAN DEVELOPMENTS

Nobel Prize winner Ivan Pavlov (1849–1936) showed that dogs' internal organs could be conditioned to respond to certain stimuli. This led Russian physicians of the early 1900s to form the hypothesis that health can be affected in response to external stimuli. This concept became known as "reflex therapy": physician Vladimir Behterev (1857–1957) coined the term "reflexology" in 1917. Physician-researchers of the time believed that an organ experienced illness because it received wrong instructions from the brain. According to this theory, by interrupting such "bad" instructions, a reflex therapist could prompt the body to return to health. Influencing health through reflex action is a concept that survives in some medical practice today.

ZONE THERAPY AND BEYOND

American physician William Fitzgerald (1872–1942) launched similar ideas in the United States. Influenced by a visit to England in the early 1900s, he observed that direct pressure could produce a pain-relieving effect, and taught that the application of pressure to a finger or toe representing one of the body's ten zones could lessen pain in the corresponding body area. Dr. Fitzgerald named this zone therapy (*see box*), and some contemporary physicians accepted his theory,

In several cultures the foot is considered to be a conduit to spirituality and general wellness.

> ### WHAT IS ZONE THERAPY?
>
> Dr. William Fitzgerald's zone therapy divided the body into ten longitudinal zones that run from the top of the head down the body to the feet. There are five zones on each side of the body, each one branching off down the respective arm and encompassing one digit on the hand, and also continuing straight down the body and down the respective leg to align with a toe on the respective foot.

using it to treat illness and as an anaesthetic during minor surgery. Controversy followed within the medical community, and while it flourished for a short period, zone therapy was displaced when modern drugs and surgical procedures became prevalent.

Dr. Fitzgerald's ideas were continued in the early 20th century through the work of individuals such as Dr. Joseph Riley, his assistant, physiotherapist Eunice Ingham (1879–1974) and others, who added their own ideas to the simple ten-zone concept. Applying zone therapy's basic principles to the feet, they added three lateral lines and further detail to create a map on the feet and hands showing which pressure points correspond to different parts of body.

In 1938, Eunice Ingham wrote her ground-breaking book *Stories the Feet Can Tell*, examining the reflex response when pressure was applied to the feet. She is credited with developing and keeping alive the ideas of zone therapy and reflexology. During her travels in the US, Canada and Europe, Ingham introduced thousands of people to the practice of reflexology, and her work is continued today by her nephew Dwight Byers in "Ingham Reflexology".

Modern reflexology now flourishes throughout the world. In the UK, Doreen Bayley pursued Ingham's work, while Hanne Marquarett continues the practice in Germany. Father Josef Eugster, a Jesuit parish priest in Taiwan, prompted a revival of the ancient Chinese traditions of foot-work in Asia during the 1980s.

HOW REFLEXOLOGY WORKS

Reflexologists use a series of pressure techniques to stimulate specific reflex areas on the feet and hands with the intention of invoking a beneficial response in other parts of the body. Reflexology maps (*see pages 16–23*) show the various reflex areas and their corresponding body parts. This mirror image of the body in the feet and hands helps reflexologists and self-help practitioners alike easily target the correct part of foot or hand on which to work.

Pressure sensors in the feet communicate instantly with the brain, internal organs and other body parts because of ancient survival needs: in extreme danger, when a reaction of fight or flight is necessary, the feet must be prepared to participate in defending or fleeing. They do this by processing environmental information gathered through pressure sensors in the soles, which helps the body determine optimal fuel and oxygen levels. The need to run, for example, requires more oxygen than

The feet act as self-tuners for the rest of the body: movements of the feet stimulate the whole system.

walking; feet ready to flee need different levels of fuel and oxygen than feet preparing to fight. So pressure signals from the soles tell the brain whether the body is standing, sitting or lying down, which helps it ascertain whether blood-sugar, oxygen, muscle-contraction and relaxation needs are currently being met. Consider what takes place during jogging. Pressure to the feet tells the brain that the jogger is running. The body adjusts its organs to provide adequate energy. Over time, a jogger's body becomes conditioned to work better. Reflexology is weightless jogging, exercising similar pressure receptors without the demands of standing and weight-bearing. For example, a single nerve travels from the centre of

the big toe to the part of the brain responsible for controlling movement, respiration and cardiac acceleration. So pressure applied to the centre of the big toe, the pituitary gland reflex area, triggers a revival response.

HOW ZONES WORK

Zone theory (*see pages 12–13*) established that the body can be divided into ten longitudinal zones running from the top of the head to the toes, and that all parts of a zone are connected. Tension in one part of the zone affects every part. By working any point of the zones, the hands and feet can release the tension and restore equilibrium to the entire zone and so to the body. Three lateral lines are also used by reflexologists to dissect the body, at the shoulders, diaphragm and waist, and in the same proportions on the soles of the feet or palms of the hands. These help pinpoint more precisely which part of the foot or hand to target with reflexology: the big toe or thumb corresponding to the head, the pelvis surrounding the heels and so on. The foot or hand thus becomes a three-dimensional map of the body.

HOW REFLEXES WORK

Imagine stepping on a nail. In response to the challenge to the sole of the foot, a reflexive action occurs through-out the body — muscular action withdraws the foot from the nail and the body experiences an adrenaline surge as well as changes in balance and internal organ function. Reflexology works on the same principle — it all happens reflexively throughout the nervous system.

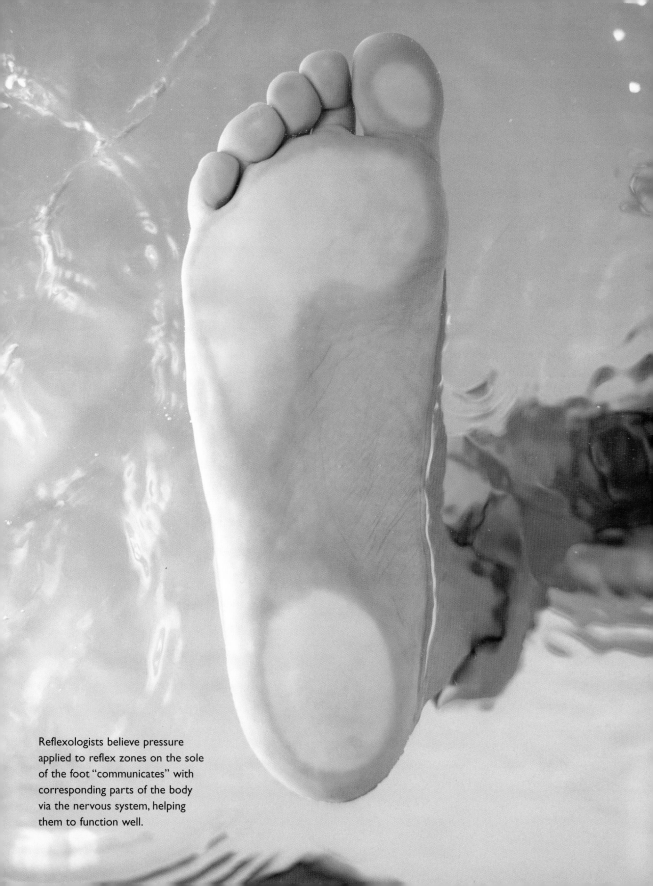

Reflexologists believe pressure
applied to reflex zones on the sole
of the foot "communicates" with
corresponding parts of the body
via the nervous system, helping
them to function well.

FOOT REFLEXOLOGY MAPS

Reflex areas on the feet form "maps" that approximate to the body's anatomy, with areas on the toes and heels, for example, reflecting the head and lower back respectively. Some reflex areas overlap, which is indicated by broken lines.

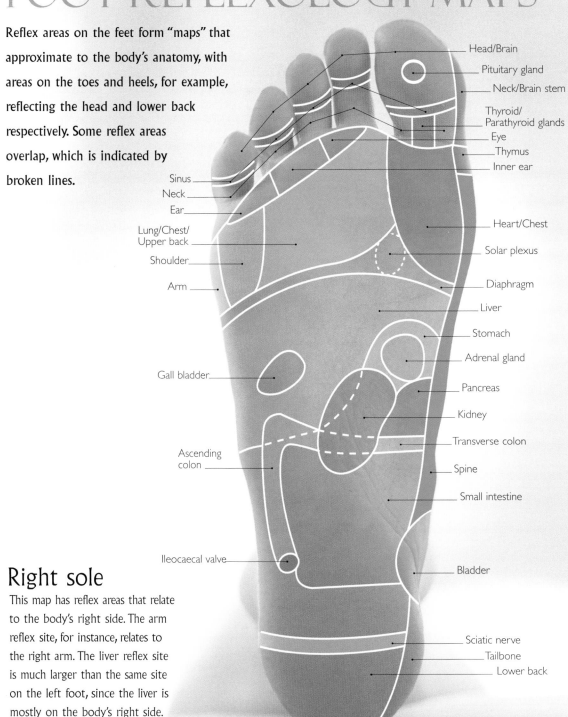

Head/Brain
Pituitary gland
Neck/Brain stem
Thyroid/
Parathyroid glands
Eye
Thymus
Inner ear

Sinus
Neck
Ear
Lung/Chest/
Upper back
Shoulder
Arm

Heart/Chest
Solar plexus
Diaphragm
Liver
Stomach
Adrenal gland
Pancreas
Kidney
Transverse colon
Spine
Small intestine

Gall bladder

Ascending
colon

Ileocaecal valve

Bladder

Sciatic nerve
Tailbone
Lower back

Right sole

This map has reflex areas that relate to the body's right side. The arm reflex site, for instance, relates to the right arm. The liver reflex site is much larger than the same site on the left foot, since the liver is mostly on the body's right side.

Left sole

Reflex areas on the left foot relate to the body's left side. The heart, stomach and pancreas reflex sites are much larger than those on the right foot map — reflecting the fact that these organs are situated on the left side of the body.

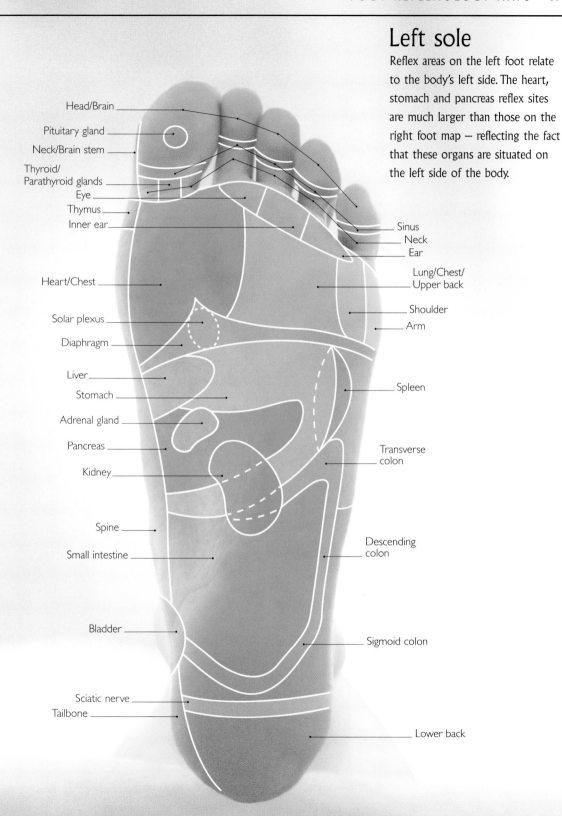

Head/Brain

Pituitary gland

Neck/Brain stem

Thyroid/
Parathyroid glands

Eye

Thymus

Inner ear

Heart/Chest

Solar plexus

Diaphragm

Liver

Stomach

Adrenal gland

Pancreas

Kidney

Spine

Small intestine

Bladder

Sciatic nerve

Tailbone

Sinus

Neck

Ear

Lung/Chest/
Upper back

Shoulder

Arm

Spleen

Transverse
colon

Descending
colon

Sigmoid colon

Lower back

Top of left foot

The reflex areas shown relate to the left side of the body. To orientate yourself, the spine reflex area lies on the inside of the foot and the shoulder reflex area on the outside. The reflex areas for the lung, chest, breast and upper back is represented as one area. However, in the same way as the chest and lungs lie "behind" the back, so the chest and lungs reflex areas actually lie behind the back reflex area.

Inside foot

This view shows how the spine reflex area runs along the inside of the foot. The neck is represented at the big toe, the area between the shoulder blades in the ball of the foot, the lower back at the arch, and the tailbone at the base of the heel.

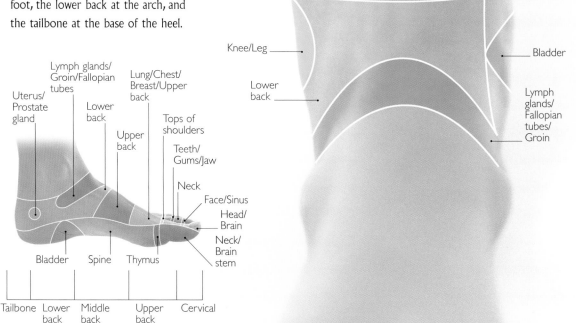

Head/Brain

Neck

Neck/Brain stem

Tops of shoulders

Thymus

Spine

Upper back

Waistline

Bladder

Lymph glands/ Fallopian tubes/ Groin

Face/Sinus

Teeth/Gums/Jaw

Arm

Lung/Chest/ Breast/ Upper back

Elbow

Knee/Leg

Lower back

Uterus/ Prostate gland

Lymph glands/ Groin/Fallopian tubes

Lower back

Upper back

Bladder

Spine

Thymus

Lung/Chest/ Breast/Upper back

Tops of shoulders

Teeth/ Gums/Jaw

Neck

Face/Sinus

Head/ Brain

Neck/ Brain stem

Tailbone

Lower back

Middle back

Upper back

Cervical

SPINAL AREA

Top of right foot

On the top of the right foot are reflex areas relating to the right side of the body, such as the right arm and leg. A point halfway down each foot is known as the "waistline". The upper back and its organs are mapped above this point, and the lower back and the internal organs it encases are below this guideline. The lymph glands and the groin reflex areas wrap around the ankle.

Head/Brain

Neck

Neck/ Brain stem

Tops of shoulders

Thymus

Spine

Upper back

Waistline

Bladder

Lymph glands/ Fallopian tubes/ Groin

Face/Sinus

Teeth/Gums/Jaw

Lung/Chest/ Breast/Upper back

Arm

Elbow

Knee/Leg

Lower back

Outside foot

The reflex area for the top of the shoulders runs across the toes, with the areas corresponding to the arm and elbow at the side of the foot. The reflex areas for the reproductive organs and for the sciatic nerve and hip, which curve round the ankle bone, can be clearly seen in this view.

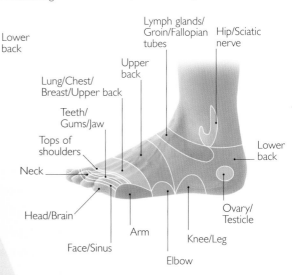

Lymph glands/ Groin/Fallopian tubes

Hip/Sciatic nerve

Upper back

Lung/Chest/ Breast/Upper back

Teeth/ Gums/Jaw

Tops of shoulders

Neck

Head/Brain

Face/Sinus

Arm

Elbow

Knee/Leg

Lower back

Ovary/ Testicle

HAND REFLEXOLOGY MAPS

Just as the hands and feet are shaped differently, so too are their respective reflexology maps. One major difference, for instance, is that the reflex areas for the head and neck are much larger on the fingers than on the toes.

Left palm

The reflex areas on the left palm relate to the left side of the body. The spine reflex area lies on the inside, and the shoulder reflex area on the outside. The head and neck reflex areas are positioned on the fingers with the tailbone near the wrist.

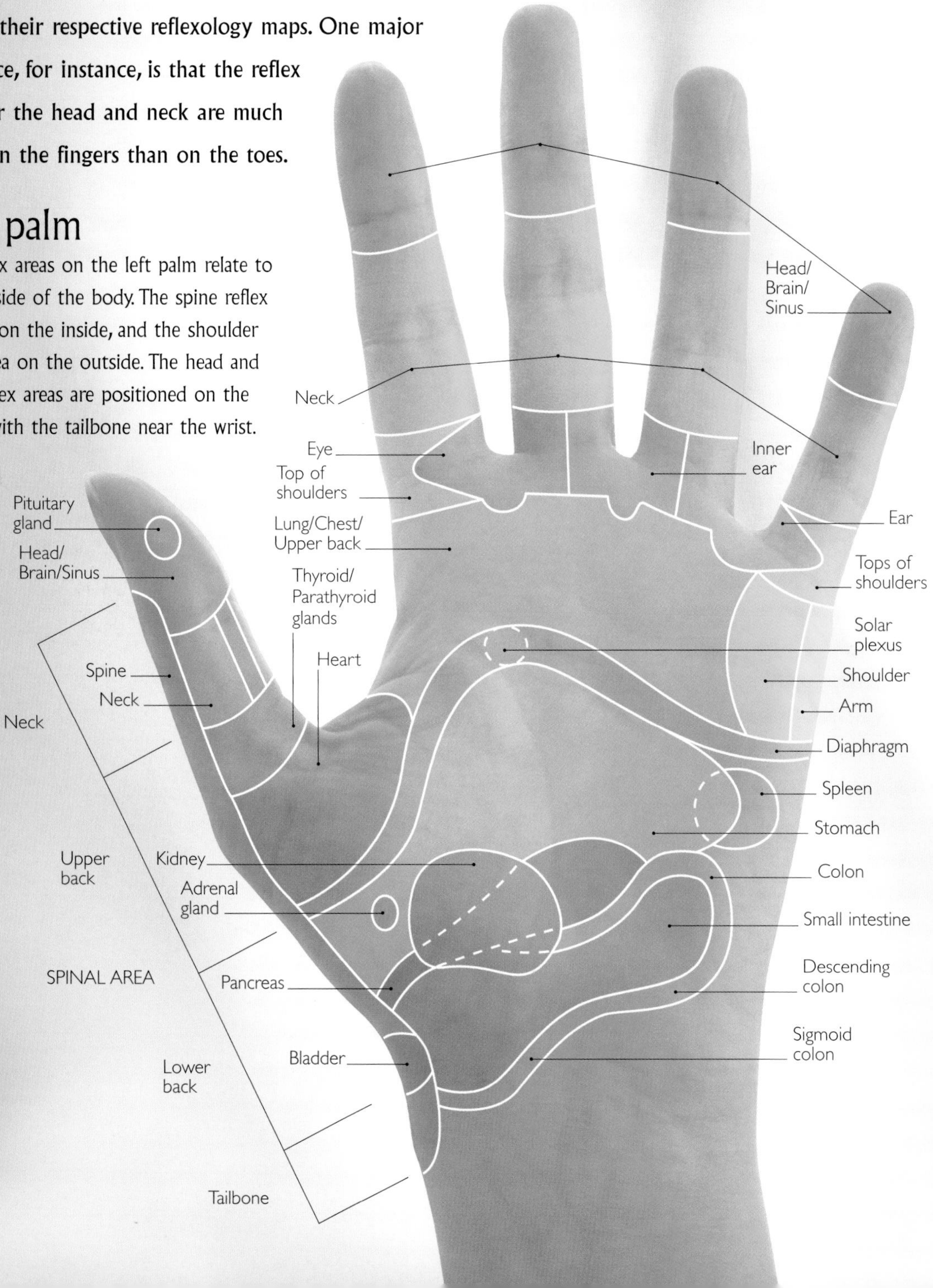

Head/ Brain/ Sinus

Neck

Eye

Top of shoulders

Lung/Chest/ Upper back

Inner ear

Ear

Tops of shoulders

Pituitary gland

Head/ Brain/Sinus

Thyroid/ Parathyroid glands

Heart

Solar plexus

Shoulder

Arm

Diaphragm

Spine

Neck

Spleen

Neck

Stomach

Upper back

Kidney

Colon

Adrenal gland

Small intestine

SPINAL AREA

Pancreas

Descending colon

Lower back

Bladder

Sigmoid colon

Tailbone

Right palm

Reflex areas on the right palm relate to the right side of the body. Mirroring the way the two sides of the body have different internal organs, there are key differences between the reflexology maps for the right and left hands. The liver, for instance, has a reflex area only on the right palm.

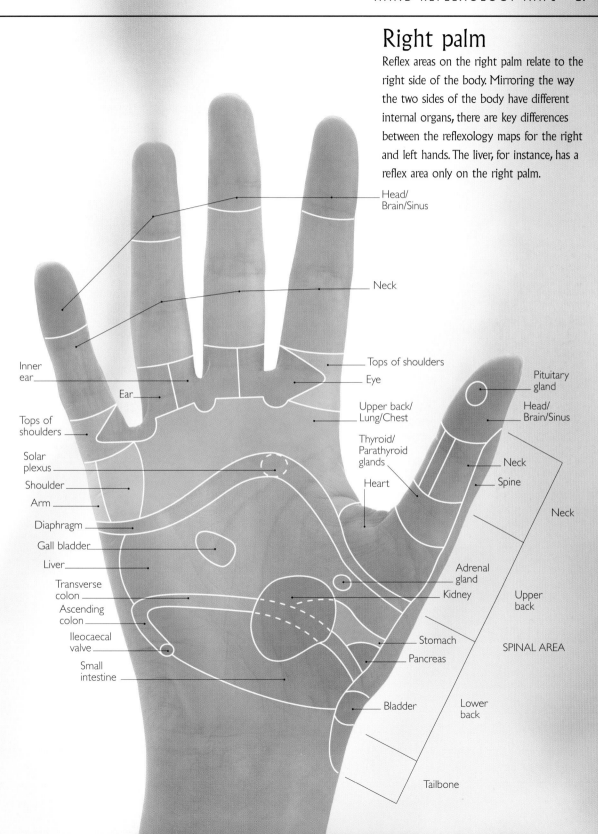

Head/Brain/Sinus

Neck

Inner ear

Ear

Tops of shoulders

Solar plexus

Shoulder

Arm

Diaphragm

Gall bladder

Liver

Transverse colon

Ascending colon

Ileocaecal valve

Small intestine

Tops of shoulders

Eye

Upper back/Lung/Chest

Thyroid/Parathyroid glands

Heart

Adrenal gland

Kidney

Stomach

Pancreas

Bladder

Pituitary gland

Head/Brain/Sinus

Neck

Spine

Neck

Upper back

SPINAL AREA

Lower back

Tailbone

Top of left hand

The top of the left hand features a series of banded reflex areas, representing the left-hand side of the body from the left side of the head to the left knee. Reflex areas for the lymph glands, groin and fallopian tubes encircle the wrist.

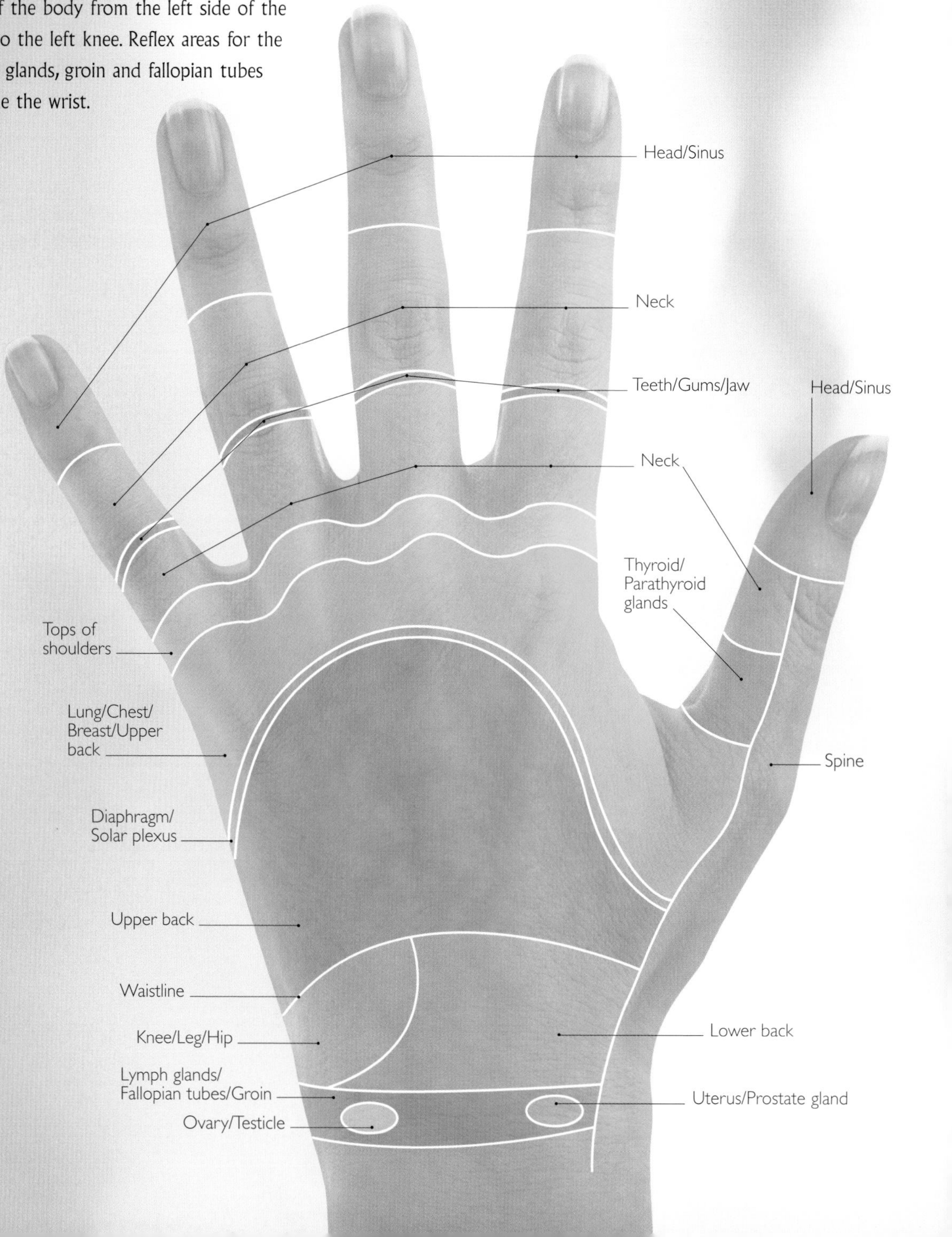

Head/Sinus

Neck

Teeth/Gums/Jaw

Head/Sinus

Neck

Thyroid/
Parathyroid
glands

Tops of
shoulders

Lung/Chest/
Breast/Upper
back

Spine

Diaphragm/
Solar plexus

Upper back

Waistline

Knee/Leg/Hip

Lower back

Lymph glands/
Fallopian tubes/Groin

Ovary/Testicle

Uterus/Prostate gland

Top of right hand

To orientate yourself, the reflex areas on the right hand relate to body's right side. At the base of the hand's long bones, is an invisible point – the "waistline". The upper back reflex area is above this point and the areas for the lower back, hips and the internal organs they encase are below it.

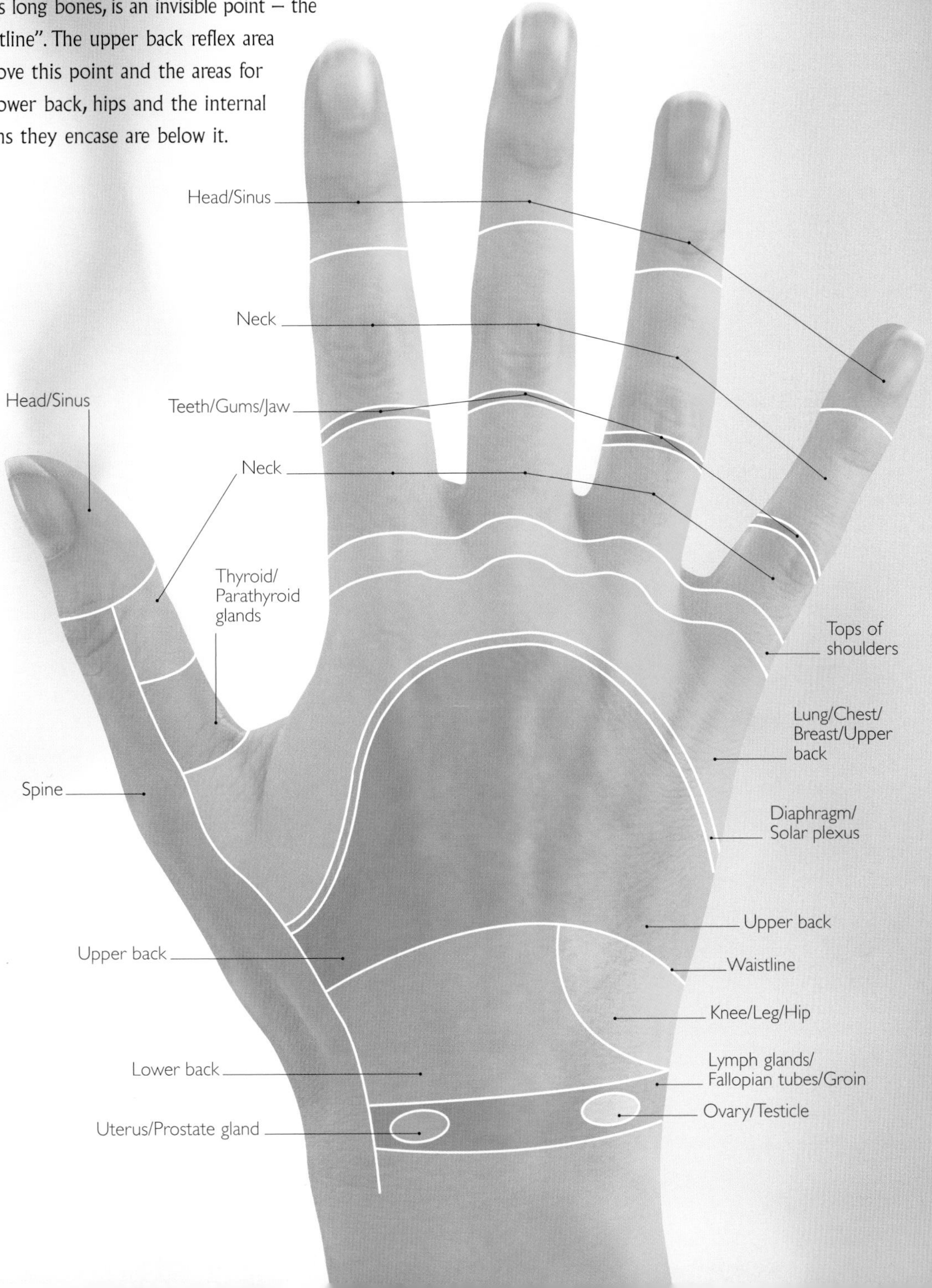

Head/Sinus

Neck

Head/Sinus

Teeth/Gums/Jaw

Neck

Thyroid/
Parathyroid
glands

Tops of
shoulders

Lung/Chest/
Breast/Upper
back

Spine

Diaphragm/
Solar plexus

Upper back

Waistline

Upper back

Knee/Leg/Hip

Lower back

Lymph glands/
Fallopian tubes/Groin

Uterus/Prostate gland

Ovary/Testicle

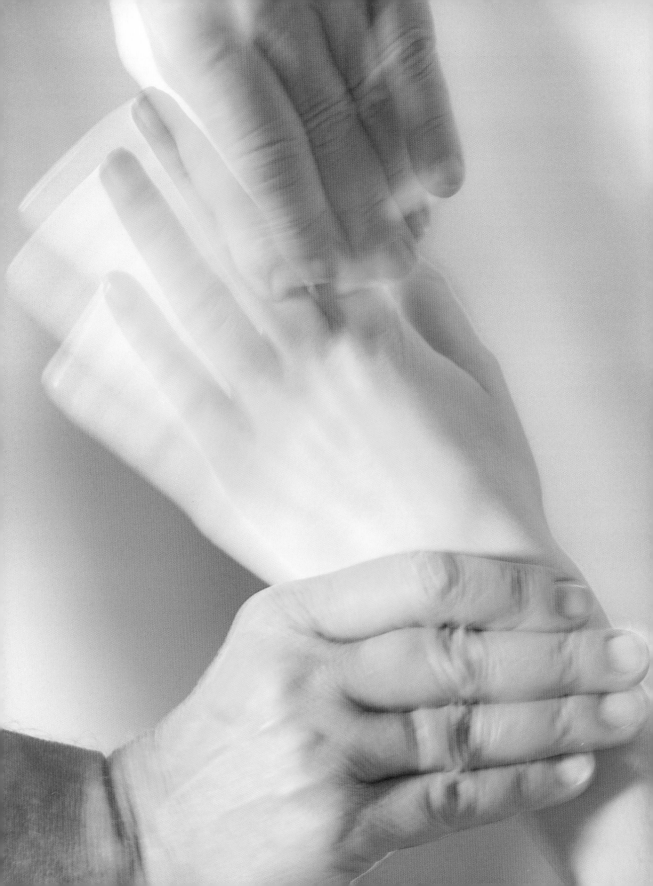

BENEFITS OF REFLEXOLOGY

Everyone can benefit enormously from reflexology.

Whether you visit a professional, practise on

yourself or have a friend apply the techniques,

studies cited in this chapter suggest that

reflexology can help relax you, alleviate symptoms

of certain disorders and generally improve your

quality of life. As well as explaining the benefits

of reflexology, this chapter also answers the most

frequently asked questions, tells you how to choose

a professional reflexologist and outlines what to

expect during a consultation.

WHY DO PEOPLE USE REFLEXOLOGY?

Of the many reasons for choosing this therapy, most people come to reflexology work because it offers a safe, effective, natural, easily available and simple-to-use treatment option for a variety of health problems. Some are attracted to the therapy because it is non-invasive and drug-free: others like the fact that it is easy to learn and to apply – self-help work can be carried out anywhere and anytime. Worldwide, people are discovering that reflexology may help treat the root causes of many health concerns, ease day-to-day stresses and relieve the impact of past injury or illness. It also presents a gentle opportunity to offer the gift of touch, to reach out and show a loved one you care.

A common thread among these benefits is the opportunity that reflexology offers for easing stress, which is thought to be a major factor in 80 per cent of illness and a contributing factor in the other 20 per cent. Applying pressure to the hands and feet simultaneously elicits general relaxation while also relaxing a targeted area. Stress researcher Hans Selye (1907–82) noted in 1956 that it is not simply stress itself, but prolonged exposure to stress, that causes wear and tear on the body. Reflex work breaks up patterns of repeated stress by treating the body to an experience apart from the mundane and everyday. One application interrupts stress; further sessions condition change to take place; and ongoing application teaches the body to operate more effectively.

Reflexology offers an opportunity to take a break from the stress of everyday life. Putting one's feet up and taking a few minutes out is effective in itself – aching hands and feet make everyday life miserable – but reflexology techniques amplify these effects.

Injury to any part of the body stresses the whole system. Pain is a stressor. Reflexology, however, releases endorphins, the body's natural pain-relieving chemicals. It also helps the body to adapt to injury. An injured shoulder, for example, prompts the whole body to hold itself differently. As reflexology de-stresses the entire body with the injured shoulder, it allows the best possible accommodation of injury. Post-injury reflex therapy encourages flexibility and motion. It exercises the building blocks of dexterity and walking, enabling muscles, tendons, ligaments and joints to use their full range of movement and ensuring maximum mobility through into old age.

WHY CHOOSE REFLEXOLOGY?

It offers a natural, drug-free treatment option for a variety of health problems	The therapy can be used to reduce pain
Reflexology can be used to aid recovery from injury, particularly injury to the feet or hands	Reflexology helps to maintain manual dexterity and locomotive abilities
It offers a non-intrusive way of expressing love or care for someone, benefiting the giver and recipient alike	The therapy can be used to maintain good health in a preventive way
It helps to ease over-used, tired feet and hands	Reflexology promotes general relaxation
	It releases endorphins, the body's "feel-good" chemicals

Your questions answered

Can reflexology help me with my health problem?

This is an impossible question to answer. There are many factors involved in healing, such as how long you've had the ailment, how severe the problem is and whether or not you have other health issues. That said, however, in our reflexology work we have often been amazed at the ability of the therapy to resolve health concerns. It's worth giving reflexology a try: whether you solve the problem or not, you are helping by taking positive steps to look after your health.

Which is more effective, hand reflexology or foot reflexology?

This is a matter of ongoing debate. Some people enjoy work on their hands, while others prefer to have their feet manipulated. Occupation can play a role in preferences: those who stand or walk all day tend to enjoy foot-work, while someone who spends time at a keyboard may prefer hand-work. Generally, foot reflexology is considered more effective because the foot is more sensitive for being encased in shoes all day. One could also argue that the feet play a more vital role in survival and so are more directly wired by the nervous system to

There are benefits to both hand and foot reflexology: foot-work is generally considered more effective as the feet are often highly sensitive, but hand-work has its own distinct advantages.

Whether you solve your health problem or not, you can gain positive support from knowing you are taking active steps to look after your health.

respond to the application of pressure techniques. The hands do, however, have unique qualities that give them their own distinct advantages: the hand is more readily accessible for self-help techniques and so may be a more effective place to apply pressure techniques simply because one is able to apply them more often. For those seeking to regain function of the hands or to maintain an independent lifestyle, hand reflexology work more effectively helps maintain or regain the ability to button, zip and manipulate objects.

Which is better, self-help or having someone else working on me?

The advantage of having someone else work on you is that you get to sit back and do nothing, gaining an increased feeling of relaxation. Self-help work, however, is convenient for frequent reflexology applications, which may be necessary if your goal is to ameliorate a chronic health concern.

Can I hurt myself?

Reflexology is very, very safe. But, like any activity involving the body, if pushed to the extreme, excessive pressure could cause bruising. There may also be an overall body response to reflexology work (a sensation of flu-like symptoms, such as achiness and tiredness) as the body attempts to release accumulated toxins. This should pass within one hour.

REFLEXOLOGY FOR EVERYONE

Whatever your occupation, age or current state of health, reflexology has something to offer you. For all stages of life, this healing therapy aims to help your body to maintain health, enhance your quality of life, meet specific health needs and relieve stress in a very pleasant way.

BABIES

Many reflexologists find babies uniquely responsive to gentle reflexology treatment. Rubbing the ear reflex area on travelling infants' feet prior to take-off or landing, for example, quickly and effectively rids the infant of the pain such experiences usually bring. A friend's baby was fussing during a visit and she asked us for help. A few gentle presses to the solar plexus reflex area of the foot calmed the infant. "Why don't we learn how to do that?" her husband asked. In this book you will find simple self-help tactics, like this one, to deal with many common infant health issues, such as colic, diarrhoea and sleep problems (*see pages 118–19*).

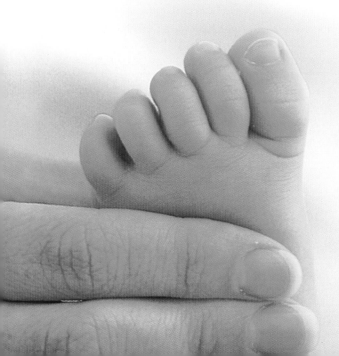

CHILDREN

Enduring images of warm person-to-person contact emerge from stories about reflexology use with young children. One woman is called "Foot" rather than "Auntie" by her two-year-old niece, who remembers and relates to her foot reflexology work. Another client had not forgotten his mother's work on his feet at bedtime every night as a child, even though 40 years had passed.

One five-year-old, during a journey, insisted on returning home for "his" golf ball. The parents learnt that he had acquired the habit of copying his childminder's reflexology golf-ball technique (*see pages 50–51*). While she used it to relieve her sinus headaches, the child had adopted it to ease his migraine headaches. The value of empowering a child to affect his or her body through a tool such as reflexology is beyond measure. How better to engender self-reliance than to give the child a means to communicate with his or her body? The application of self-help techniques allows the child an opportunity to interact with his or her "owies", as one two-year-old puts it. Children's natural curiosity and innate ability to learn create a unique role for reflexology in a child's life. The ability to "play" with one's hands and feet for benefit does not escape the notice of children.

Reflexology provides a wonderful way to connect with the children in your life. This may be especially valuable when watching a child experience illness, and it is at such times that many parents turn to reflexology to bolster conventional medical care. Use this book to help with childhood aches and pains (*see pages 118–19*).

OLDER PEOPLE

A succession of pension-age clients began requesting Friday appointments with us: their reasons soon became clear when one asked for "the tune-up". He explained that another client had told all his friends about how reflexology helped his love life and made weekends more fun. This hints at the improved quality of life that reflexology may offer pensioners. Ageing presents unique challenges and an increased need for solutions to special concerns. Whether you wish to ameliorate the physical effects of ageing, such as aching joints and incontinence, or simply to reach out and touch someone older who has limited access to physical contact, use some of the ideas in this book to help you (*see pages 122–23*).

PEOPLE WITH PHYSICAL DISABILITIES

When a serious degenerative disease prevented one of our clients operating the television remote control, it robbed him of his last form of entertainment. Reflexology sessions, however, helped him recover the use of his thumb and regain control of the television. Reflexology can be used to provide special stimulation for special people. Without pressure to the soles of the feet, for example, the associated muscles, nerves and bones may degenerate, and so, for those who spend a great deal of time in a wheelchair, reflexology provides welcome sensory stimulation. For those trying to maintain function in the hands, applying hand-work can boost manipulative skills. In our work, we have also seen reflexology increase muscle tone and have a positive impact on internal organs. As well as helpful general foot and hand workouts (*see pages 68–117*), you will find in this book techniques to target a range of health concerns (*see pages 130–53*).

THOSE WITH SERIOUS ILLNESS

A friend called not too long ago to ask for referral to a reflexologist in her city. She wanted help for her once-estranged sister, who had just been diagnosed with cancer and had but a short time to live. Instead, we told her how she could use reflexology herself to work with her sister. She later wrote to tell us how much it had meant to both of them. Reflexology, while offering the potential to counter pain and help ease the symptoms of specific conditions, is perhaps as useful to giver as recipient in that it provides an opportunity to offer a loved one tangible support during a difficult time. In such circumstances, it provides an extremely valuable extra measure of care that goes beyond what a professional can provide. Relish the chance to reach out and make a difference, and to empower yourself as well as ease the pain of a loved one with the techniques that target specific health problems (*see pages 130–53*).

PREGNANT WOMEN

As she was being rolled into the delivery room, our niece insisted that someone get her golf ball for use as a reflexology tool during delivery. The nurses were surprised when she delivered so quickly and easily. Reflexology use is increasing among medical personnel involved in pregnancy and childbirth, and studies vouch for its efficacy. In *The Effects of Reflexology on Labour Outcome* (UK, 1989), Dr. Gowri Motha and Jane McGrath found that pregnant women who completed a course of ten sessions of reflexology experienced benefits in labour outcomes

Benefits in labour perceived as outstanding were experienced by pregnant women who had completed a set course of ten reflexology treatments.

perceived as outstanding. Some had labour times of only 2–3 hours: those aged 20–25 had an average first-stage labour time of 5–6 hours, an average second stage of 16 minutes and a third stage of 7 minutes. This compares well against the textbook average figures of 16–24 hours for a first stage of labour, and 1–2 hours for the second stage. Gabriella Bering Liisberg claimed in her 1989 study,

Easier Births Using Reflexology, that 90 per cent of women who chose reflexology as an alternative to painkilling drugs or drugs aimed at inducing and stimulating labour stated that reflexology had helped reduce their pain.

Whether you wish to use pain-relief techniques in labour, or simply want to soothe the symptoms and discomforts associated with pregnancy and labour, such as oedema and an aching lower back, that can make the 40 weeks of pregnancy uncomfortable, this book provides you with the resources (*see pages 120–21 and 130–53*).

IN THE WORKPLACE

Our client Sue considered leaving the teaching profession due to sore feet – she could no longer stand comfortably in front of a class all day. Once she became aware of reflexology techniques for breaking up patterns of stress, however, she invented a solution to her problem. Several times a day, she walked barefoot on the rounded sticks used by her elementary-school music students.

Reflexology is particularly beneficial for those in jobs that require long hours of standing or walking, such as teaching, nursing, hairdressing, waiting at tables

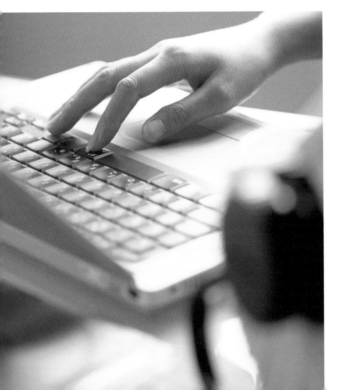

and sales professions. It offers an opportunity to interrupt the stress of standing and of over-using one part of the body by providing a break in routine. It also helps establish new patterns of using the body and a more relaxed state of being, as, to paraphrase stress researcher Hans Selye, it is not just the stress that creates the problem, but the continuity of that stress.

For the same reasons, those who work long hours at keyboards often use hand reflexology to relieve symptoms caused by overuse of this part of the body. Try the self-help techniques for hands and feet, and for those in the office and on the move (*see pages 124–29*).

THOSE WITH MENTAL HEALTH NEEDS

At a British walk-in health clinic for people with mental health problems, a reflexologist and a counsellor worked with 74 people during 1996–97, with 49 receiving reflexology and 25 receiving counselling. All but two of the clients undergoing reflexology reported an increased level of relaxation and a decrease in feelings of anxiety. Release of tension through being able to talk led to a greater feeling of relaxation, alleviating headaches and improving sleep. Such studies highlight the important role reflexology and other one-to-one complementary therapies can play in helping relieve the symptoms of mental health problems. Of particular importance was that the participants developed and increased their awareness of the effects of tension, and discovered an increased ability to change that state of being. The result was an encouraging improvement in emotional status, especially where reflexology and counselling were offered in tandem.

To help replace feelings such as fear, worry and despair with more positive and fulfilling emotions, you might like to try the general foot and hand routines (*see pages 68–117*) as well as the self-help care (*see pages 124–29*).

Repetitive work such as typing, or jobs involving long hours of standing, can cause patterns of stress: reflexology can interrupt these stresses and ease associated tensions.

REFLEXOLOGY RESEARCH

For the 60 years of reflexology's modern history, reflexologists have reported success stories. Now clinical research is catching up, producing studies that note the positive benefits of reflexology, such as speedier post-operative recovery, or a decrease in symptoms associated with coronary heart disease.

Recent research has shown reflexology to be effective at encouraging the body to return to a state of natural equilibrium. An Austrian study in 1999 and a Chinese study in 1994, for example, showed respectively that kidney and bowel function of those receiving reflexology seem to be more efficient. Three Chinese trials in 1996 reported that mothers often gave birth more easily and lactated more quickly, children with cerebral palsy showed improved growth rates and patients receiving reflexology demonstrated diminished levels of free radicals.

HELPING TO TACKLE SYMPTOMS

A Chinese study in 1998 revealed that, for those patients receiving foot reflexology sessions, symptoms of chest distress, coronary heart disease and angina dispersed and blood-pressure levels dropped. Foot reflexology helped patients pass kidney and ureter stones faster (according to a 1996 Chinese study) and less painfully (as reported in a Danish trial in 1993). In a 1994 Swiss study, some post-operative patients receiving reflexology work exhibited signs of enhanced kidney and bowel activity and demonstrated a decreased need for medication when compared with control groups, as did some mothers who gave birth using reflexology for pain relief. Research conducted for specific conditions,

including sinusitis (US, 2000), headaches (Denmark, 1997), toothaches (China, 1994), PMS (*Obstetrics and Gynecology*, 1993), amenorrhoea (China, 1996), male sexual dysfunction (China, 1996), hyperlipidaemia (high levels of fat in the blood: China, 1996), constipation (China, 1994) and multiple sclerosis (UK, 1997), reflected a reduction in symptoms for patients receiving reflexology work.

A SAFER OPTION?

Various research studies in China between 1993 and 1998 suggested that reflexology may be safer than conventional medical treatment in alleviating the symptoms of certain conditions, such as uroschesis (the retention of urine following surgery), dyspepsia, neuro-dermatitis, leukopaenia (an abnormally low white blood cell count) and coronary heart disease. There was evidence in other Chinese trials during the same period to suggest that reflexology combined with conventional treatment could improve the effectiveness of medication for diabetes, kidney infection and infantile pneumonia.

Most importantly, perhaps, studies have concluded that reflexology can bring a marked improvement in quality of life. In 1995 it was reported in the UK that people with Alzheimer's disease who were receiving reflexology work exhibited alleviated symptoms of restlessness and wandering alongside a reduction in stiffness and arthritis. A study in 1997 by Peta Trousdale and Andrea Uphoff-Chmielnik established positive results for people with mental health problems. Those receiving reflexology work exhibited increased relaxation, decreased anxiety, eased headaches and improved sleep patterns. In many cases, people reported that positive, fulfilling emotions replaced fear, worry and despair.

A Swiss trial in 1994 found that post-operative patients receiving foot reflexology exhibited a reduced need for medication.

REFLEXOLOGY IN MEDICAL CARE

In recent years, some conventional medical practitioners have welcomed reflexology as a treatment able to complement their own practice. Some midwives and obstetricians regard the therapy as a safe, natural and non-invasive way to care for mothers in labour. Doctors may use it in hospitals to support post-operative recovery and intensive care, and reflexology can play a valuable role in palliative care.

OBSTETRICS AND GYNAECOLOGY

Nurses and midwives in obstetric and gynaecological units have embraced reflexology to help relieve labour pains and to resolve complications. Reflexology can be used to induce labour – indeed, some nurses and midwives on the website www.babyworld.co.uk suggest it may be more effective than rupturing the membranes – and to increase the strength and efficacy of contractions. Reflexology can also be used to calm contractions that are too painful, or regulate contractions that are sporadic. Some practitioners claim that reflexology can reduce the length of a labour or offer patients a welcome rest, or even sleep, between contractions during a long birth. In the third stage of childbirth, reflexology can be used to help expel a retained placenta, and also help relieve urinary retention after delivery. Such results are reported by the Reflexology Department of the National Maternity Hospital in Dublin, Ireland. Established in 1995 following demands by doctors, patients and midwives, it reports enormous benefits across women's services in hospitals: as well as for obstetrics, treatment is given for ante- and post-partum depression, endometriosis and PMS.

REFLEXOLOGY IN HOSPITALS

Medical use of reflexology is not restricted to women's healthcare services. It is included in programmes at several surgical departments of Columbia University in New York City. The Columbia Integrative Medicine

Program of the Department of Surgery has established that reflexology is an ideal therapy for use in intensive care units or for patients immediately after surgery, since reflexology techniques applied to the feet leave more sensitive parts of the body undisturbed.

Reflexology also plays a important role at the Complementary Cardiac Care Unit at Columbia-Presbyterian Medical Center in New York City. Here, the inclusion of complementary medicine alongside conventional care has been patient-driven – many of the cardiac patients had already explored complementary therapies. The centre notes that massage and reflexology, for instance, are both popular among patients in the programme and that nearly 60 per cent of patients entering the unit use them. That is, of the 1,400 cardiac care unit patients seen here each year, 60 per cent choose to participate in complementary medicine in this way.

REFLEXOLOGY USE IN MEDICINE

Medical facilities and hospices report using reflexology to help with the following:

Obstetrics and gynaecology, particularly during childbirth and its complications

Post-operative care

Patient support classes

Palliative care for cancer patients

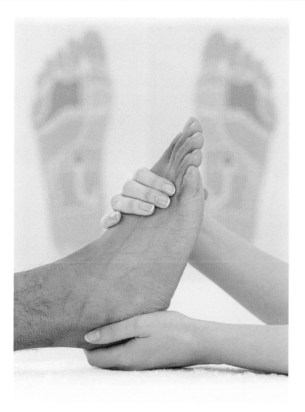

Increasingly, reflexology work is being integrated into healthcare programmes at several hospitals, playing a role in palliative care and in post-operative treatment.

PATIENT SUPPORT

In some healthcare establishments in the US, reflexology classes are offered to patients, educating them in self-care strategies that may help to ease their medical problems. Reflexology classes for people with incontinence, for example, are held at Suburban Hospital in Bethesda, Maryland. Reflexology classes are also taught at Southpoint Hospital in Chagrin Falls, Ohio, and Avera Queen of Peace Hospital's Wellness Center in South Dakota. Some practitioners are interested in the potential emotional and preventive support such self-help therapies may offer. One such practitioner is Dr. Mehmet Oz, co-founder of the Complementary Cardiac Care Unit of the Columbia-Presbyterian Medical Center in New York City. He is eager to learn how complementary therapies such as reflexology might help alleviate the post-surgical impact on patients of depression, anxiety, pain and infection, stating that "…as allopathic clinicians, physicians felt that the emotional, palliative and/or preventive care requested by patients were areas that surgeons were not well trained to provide."

PALLIATIVE CARE

Reflexology also increasingly plays a role in the palliative care of cancer patients. In the UK, reflexology is included at complementary therapy centres within cancer units at Charing Cross Hospital, Hammersmith Hospital, the Harley Street Clinic and Lister Hospital. And outside such centres, cancer support groups, such as Cancer BACUP Cancer Support Service and the Hampshire County Council Cancer Care Society provide reflexology services, information and referrals to reflexologists. But the giving of reflexology treatments is not confined to medical staff. Concerned family members and volunteers eager to express their care through touch-work offer reflexology to loved ones alongside paid professionals in cancer units and hospices.

Across the UK, the provision of reflexology services has grown to meet hospice goals, which are to provide dignity, choices and control for each patient and family. Specific aims for reflexology work here include improving a patient's quality of life, offering practical ways to cope with life-threatening illness, providing comfort and enhancing both the patient's and the carer's sense of physical, emotional and spiritual well-being, and all while helping to control the symptoms of specific diseases and alleviating general symptoms including pain and anxiety.

The *American Cancer Society Journal* found that one third of cancer patients used reflexology as an alternative medical approach.

SUCCESS STORIES

The world of reflexology is alive with success stories recounted by practitioners and patients alike. Such anecdotal evidence attests to the willingness of reflexology patients to participate in the healing process, a factor that may be vital for the efficacy of complementary therapies.

Stories of success illustrate the benefits of reflexology, above all, its ability to elicit a relaxation response in body and mind in a natural, drug-free way, and release endorphins, the body's "feel-good" chemicals, possibly the best way to relieve stress. Reflexology treatments help our clients survive the demands of high-pressure jobs, busy family lives and active athletic pastimes.

Reflexology is also highly valued by patients and practitioners as a means of triggering the body to respond to particular ailments, and by rebalancing body, mind and emotions, to maintain health by preventing medical conditions arising or worsening. There is evidence to indicate that some reflexology techniques even reduce the need for medication, or help medicines work more effectively. Reflexology thus offers a means of interacting with and gaining a sense of control over the body – and the knowledge that one can have a positive effect on one's own health can only provide an emotional uplift.

On a practical level, many success stories acclaim reflexology for aiding recovery from the pain of injury, particularly of the feet and hands, and even for helping the body recover from past injuries. In easing overused hands and feet, reflexology is also thought to prevent injury occurring and to help maintain manual dexterity and mobility into later life.

Case studies
The relaxation response
It is not uncommon for our clients to fall asleep during a reflexology session. Indeed, some choose to use reflexology for the relaxing effect it prompts over the whole body. The benefits of such overall relaxation are hard to measure. One client, perceiving his stress level as high, regards reflexology as having the ability to "save his life"; he rightly welcomes the break in a stressful workday that his reflexology sessions provide as an opportunity for his body to rest and heal itself.

As she walked into the office for her session, the client asked what the noise was. "It's your husband," Kevin replied. Her husband, a high-powered lawyer, had fallen asleep during his session and was snoring loudly.

Injury-repair
It had been 40 years since the high-school coach had sent our client back into the game with what turned out to be a broken heelbone. Our client was still aware of the injury, however, as he travelled for business, rushing through airports, or played a game of tennis during his leisure time. "When I see the doctor, I get a prescription," he reported to us. "When I see you reflexologists, I simply feel better."

Easing common health problems

Life was made miserable for our client Bob by his sinus problems and sinus headaches. Medicines simply would not help his problem, and other complementary therapies didn't seem to help either. We showed Bob a simple reflexology golf-ball technique (*see page 50*), which gave him the resources to heal his problem. Bob did, however, develop a new problem: annoyance with his office colleague's sinus problems. Tired of listening to his colleague's symptoms, he gave him a golf ball and taught him the technique too. Reflexology enabled Bob not only to address his own health issues, but offer non-intrusive help to others wishing to address their own health problems.

With reflexology, Bob could not only gain control over his own state of health but help others too.

Freedom from medication

Her asthma and struggling to breathe would wake our client Susan in the middle of the night. Susan's concern was that she had become de-sensitised to her prescribed asthma medication and that it no longer offered a solution. We showed her a self-help technique to apply to the adrenal gland reflex area. She reported back that she could breathe freely again after applying the technique.

Rejuvenating the hands and feet

Her catering business kept our client Sharon on her feet for hours at a time. Tired feet and tired hands were taking their toll on her health, as were the headaches, backaches and fatigue that accompanied them. Sharon felt her overall health was going downhill. Having relieved her symptoms, reflexology sessions now gain her total devotion. She says they have changed her life.

Sharon, like many others, has extended reflexology use to her whole family. Her mother's eye problem, her daughter's whiplash injury and another daughter's tiredness have all been addressed by reflexology treatment.

Instant results

Our client was a minister's kind wife who would eat the food served to her at a parishioner's house even though it gave her extreme gastric distress. On the way to hospital following one such event, she tried a hand reflexology technique we had showed her. The driver turned round on seeing that she had relieved herself of the distress so completely.

The client reported that she appreciated not only the relief from the gastric distress, but also the relief of not having to visit casualty.

VISITING A REFLEXOLOGIST

Visiting a reflexologist is like visiting any other healthcare professional. You should expect the same professional environment and attitude from a reflexologist as from a doctor or dentist. A professional environment includes a clean, well-lit and inviting workplace. Expect to be seated on a reclining chair or perhaps a massage table, and check that the therapist ensures that your knees are supported during reflexology work. Expect to remove your shoes and socks or tights – some women may feel more comfortable wearing trousers, or should be offered a towel to cover their bare legs.

The length of a reflexology session can range from 30–45 minutes up to even an hour in length. A professional reflexologist should apply the techniques systematically and thoroughly to each foot. After finishing work on one foot, the practitioner should apply further techniques to areas that he or she considers need more work. "Desserts", or feel-good techniques, should also be applied.

Technique application should fall within your comfort level. This means it should "hurt good" if it hurts at all, and not seem threatening in any way. If you feel any discomfort, ask the reflexologist to lighten pressure, and he or she should do so.

Expect a professional reflexologist to apply sufficient and appropriate techniques to give you a sense of relaxation. You should also be given feedback as he or she carries out the session and assesses different reflex areas. In turn, he or she should also listen to your concerns and pay attention to your likes and dislikes. Favourite desserts, areas to which technique is applied and parts that you report "hurt good", should all be remembered by the reflexologist for subsequent treatments.

MASSAGE OR REFLEXOLOGY?

Reflexology is considered a science by many, but there is also an art to the craft. While there is a professional standard of practice, the specifics of the pressure techniques used can vary from individual to individual and depend on where he or she received training. The use of creams, lotions and oils is accepted by some reflexologists, while others argue that this is foot massage and not necessarily reflexology.

Questions to ask

When opting for a reflexology session, stay aware of your own tastes and keep in mind the reasons why you approached the reflexologist. Whether it is tired feet, relaxation, a health concern or another reason, make your interests known to the reflexologist. It is important to ask questions of your reflexologist to ensure you receive appropriate treatment. You might find it useful to start by thinking about some of the following questions.

Questions to ask yourself:

How do I feel after the session?

After you've tried a reflexology session, ask yourself whether you feel that your feet or hands have been thoroughly worked, your questions have been fully answered and you have been treated professionally. Finally, try to assess whether you have received your money's worth.

What physical sensations do I feel?

You should experience feelings of relaxation after a reflexology session. Some individuals feel a direct impact on their feet. Common statements include "My feet feel lighter," and "I feel as if I'm walking on pillows."

Questions to ask the reflexologist:

What training and experience do you have?

A reflexologist who has completed a course of study of 50 hours or more and who has at least a year's experience of practice will often have the training and experience you are looking for. Be aware that standards have changed over the years. Ten years ago, a weekend course was acceptable to qualify someone to practise. Someone with ten years' experience following a weekend course may be worth visiting, but a practitioner educated recently with a weekend

course but having little practical experience may not be able to provide the skilled services you require. Check your practitioner's credentials for any qualifications and membership of reflexology organisations (see page 154).

Do you provide other services or sell products?

Be aware that someone who has expanded into selling products or offering other complementary therapies may not be as experienced in giving reflexology treatment as a full-time reflexologist.

What kind of services do you provide?

Ask the reflexologist about the nature of his or her services, for example, whether the practitioner primarily works on the hands or feet. You may prefer to have your hands worked rather than your feet, perhaps depending on your occupation and your daily patterns of hand and foot use. Whether he or she offers sessions using cream, oil or lotion is another factor. The question is whether the practitioner is providing reflexology or foot massage services. You should ensure that the answer matches what you are comfortable with and what is effective for you.

How many sessions do I need in order to see results?

You should start seeing results within two or three sessions – you may notice that you feel more relaxed or that a particular health problem has eased. Be wary of any practitioner who, in your opinion, seems to pressure you into much longer courses of treatment. However, do keep in mind that the longer you have had a health problem, the longer it will be before results begin to show.

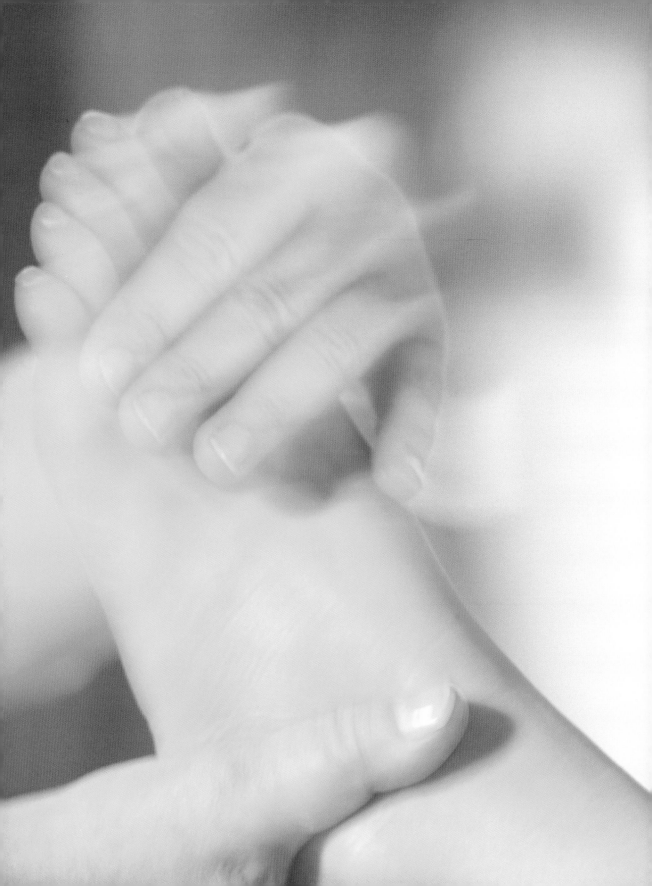

TAKING CARE OF HANDS AND FEET

With all the stresses and strains your hands and feet experience on a day-to-day basis, it's no wonder that regular reflexology sessions are such a healthy treat. In this chapter you'll find tips on using self-help tools to relax your feet and hands, as well as advice on how to break up potentially harmful "stress patterns" caused by repetitive daily activities, such as walking and typing. In this chapter we also explain what kinds of shoes you should – and should never – wear.

ANATOMY OF THE FEET AND HANDS

Humans are the only creatures on earth that walk fully upright on two legs, and with every step, each foot withstands two and a half times the weight of the body. The structure of the foot has evolved to accommodate this pressure with a complex arrangement of 26 bones, muscles, ligaments and nerves.

We often become more familiar with the anatomy of feet that cause problems than those that do their job well. But because the foot forms the body's main daily interface with the ground, each structure within it plays an important role, whether the body is walking, running or simply standing.

When we stand, the ball of the foot and the heel form a stable platform that bears the weight of the body. When we walk or run, the heel receives the initial impact. The foot then rolls forwards with the help of the longitudinal arch, while the Achilles tendon in the calf contracts to lift the heel. The weight of the body then shifts onto the ball of the foot. This includes the metatarsal arch, which runs horizontally across the foot. This structure helps to roll the foot inwards and/or outwards to adjust to changing terrain. In the final stage of a footstep, the toes propel the foot, and consequently the body, forwards in a "toe-off" action.

The enormous pressures experienced by feet daily in this repetitive unconscious action are compounded by modern inventions (such as shoes and flat surfaces), injuries and, most notably, inherited variant foot features, or "hereditary foot features". A second toe longer than its adjacent big toe is one example, and would not cause a problem for someone living a bare-footed existence. However, when faced with shoes and flat, hard modern surfaces, a long second toe can cause the centre of the foot literally to lock up. It no longer possesses the ability to help absorb the shock of each step. The result: a tight, tired foot.

The arch is also affected by hereditary factors. High and low arches form two ends of a spectrum, and the more deviation from what is considered "normal", the less effectively the structure is able to perform. Poor functioning can result in pain and deformity, such as claw-shaped hammertoes and plantar fasciitis, a localised inflammation of connective tissue. The tendency towards arthritic hands and the formation of bunions on the feet are also hereditary, the latter associated with problems including corns, pain, finding shoes that fit and difficulty in walking.

THE HANDS

Designed to perform a variety of precise, intricate tasks with their complex arrangement of 26 bones, muscles, tendons and nerves, the hands and wrists can become almost as sore and painful as the feet. The opposable thumb mankind has evolved allows us to grasp, but the repetition of grasping movements can lead to soreness in this digit. Other painful conditions include carpal tunnel syndrome, in which swollen tissue in the wrist pinches the nerve that runs through it. Because of their constant use and and susceptibility to injury, hands need care and attention. Hands, like feet, are rich in sensitive nerve endings and very receptive to reflexology.

86 per cent of the world's population experience a foot problem at some point in life.

Bones in the feet and hands

The bones of the hands and feet reflect their
different uses. The phalanges in the toes, for
example, are much shorter than those of the
fingers because the toes are only used for
balance and lift, while the fingers are used for
grip. The intricate bones of the feet are strong
enough to support the weight of the entire
body, yet light enough to move easily. The little
carpal bones of the wrist and metacarpals in
the fingers operate together as a sophisticated
set of levers with the opposable thumbs to
provide the grasping action.

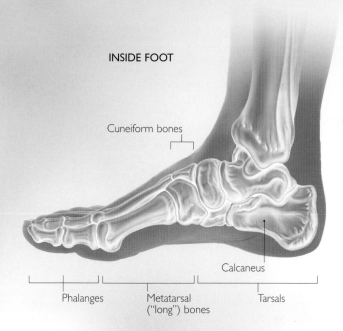

INSIDE FOOT

Cuneiform bones

Calcaneus

Phalanges

Metatarsal
("long") bones

Tarsals

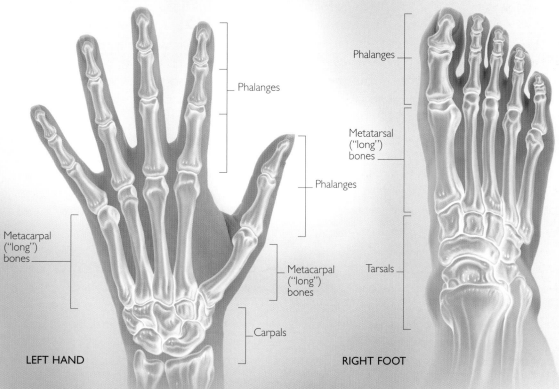

Phalanges

Phalanges

Metatarsal
("long")
bones

Metacarpal
("long")
bones

Phalanges

Metacarpal
("long")
bones

Tarsals

Carpals

LEFT HAND

RIGHT FOOT

FEET AND HANDS: AN OWNER'S MANUAL

The world is not flat, but most urban feet wouldn't know it. Cobblestone roads have given way to concrete pavements, but such modernisation of surfaces has resulted in a loss of texture and variety underfoot, and so feet tend to move in the same way, all day, every day. This repeated stress leaves the modern foot susceptible to injury. Avoid problems by combining the advice that follows for feet (and stressed hands, too) with your regular reflexology workouts.

The foot is very good at adapting itself to a set of specified demands, such as walking on smooth pavements. However, if these demands don't vary often enough, the feet, and subsequently the rest of the body, pay a price. As with all forms of exercise, underuse of any of the structures of the feet can cause them to suffer from a decline in strength, and this can create complex, often subtle, health problems. The foot can also adapt itself to stressful situations by shifting responsibility from the correct part of its anatomy onto another part that may be ill-designed for such functions. Such repetitive incorrect movement can lead to an uneven displacement of weight within the body, which results in tight, restricted muscles.

RESTORING THE FOOT'S POTENTIAL

The health of the feet can be improved simply by walking, running and standing on a variety of surfaces that stimulate different pressure sensors and allow each foot to use its full range of motion. Walking on the textured surfaces of health pathways, for example, can stimulate neglected pressure sensors in the foot and break up ingrained stress patterns. Health pathways, such as those suggested on pages 46–49, combine the benefits for the feet of the downwards pull of gravity with a variety of surface textures that challenge muscles, tendons, bones and sensors.

The foot reacts to varying terrain through its ability to move in four basic directions. The most-used directions are experienced during the heel-to-toe movement of a footstep. Two less common directions used by the feet are inwards and outwards movements. Practising these four directions gives back to the foot its full range of possible motion. The surfaces on which we walk play an important role in shock absorption, too. If these surfaces do not accept part of the shock, the body must absorb it all. The hardness of a surface determines how much shock it absorbs — hard surfaces such as concrete, asphalt or hardwood absorb little shock, while soft, yielding surfaces such as grass and sand absorb more. While it would be nice if life were a "walk on the beach", walkers today most commonly face surfaces that are hard, unyielding and unforgiving. Through health pathways, reflexology offers the chance to compensate for one's environment and so to relax the whole body.

CARING FOR THE HANDS

We must not overlook the hands. The simple exercise of gently pulling on the fingers provides a mini-holiday for digits compressed throughout the day by tapping on a keyboard. Wringing the hands can also become an opportunity to move the hands in a seldom-experienced direction. Basic exercises similar to those for the feet exist for the hands (*see pages 54–55*).

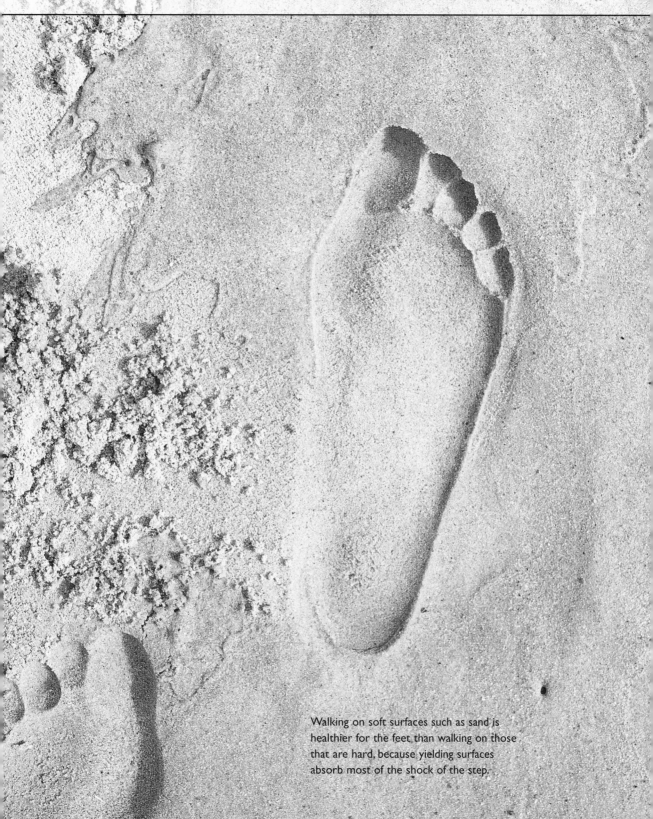

Walking on soft surfaces such as sand is
healthier for the feet than walking on those
that are hard, because yielding surfaces
absorb most of the shock of the step.

CHOOSING SHOES

On natural surfaces, the bare foot works best, but researchers have found that going barefoot is not ideal on surfaces such as concrete. With only the padding of the heel, bare feet provide no insulation against the shock of a hard surface. Therefore, the correct shoes have an enormous impact on the well-being of your feet, as well as on the rest of the body. If you follow the advice below, finding the best footwear for you will become second nature. If in doubt, remember the following maxim: do not buy or wear shoes that hurt.

Size: you may think you know your shoe size, but you may not know that the size of an adult foot can change, especially for women during pregnancy. A child's foot size changes as many as 26 times. Have your feet measured when you buy shoes, and you may find that, like most people, one foot is larger than the other. Buy for the larger foot. To ensure a proper fit, shop for shoes in the late afternoon or evening after any swelling has already occurred.

Comfort: don't buy shoes solely for their stylishness or appearance, but on how comfortable your foot feels wearing them. A poorly designed shoe could look fashionable, but if it hurts your foot, your entire body may suffer. A shoe with a high heel, for example, pitches body weight forwards onto the balls of the feet, placing a heavy demand on the wearer to maintain an awkward posture. Shoes with a pointed toe do not allow the toes to play their role in walking. A low kitten-heeled shoe provides a too-small base on which to balance and walk. Platform shoes can lead to twisted ankles, and high-tech trainers have a limited lifespan. All these shoes may look great, but could do a great deal of damage to the feet.

Bare feet

The feet act as a base for the body, holding it upright and stable. They also propel the body forwards in motion. The foot absorbs any shock incurred from movement, and disperses the body's weight evenly throughout its structures. Although walking barefoot is good on soft surfaces, hard structures may cause damage.

Sandals

This type of footwear does not have the restrictive, and often painful, toe boxes that are characteristic of other shoes. It should be noted, however, that although they may be comfortable, not all sandals have the support necessary for walking on hard surfaces, walking for long distances or running.

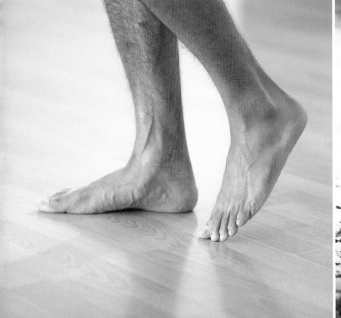

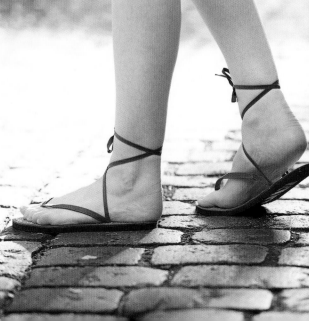

Remember, too, that even well-made shoes can become dangerous once they wear out. That favourite pair of shoes that has finally broken in may actually have broken down.

Socks: when shoe shopping, put on the type of socks or tights you would normally wear with the shoe. You should be able to lay your toes flat and wiggle them inside the shoe.

Shape: the shape of a shoe should match the shape of your foot. If the long bones and the toes — integral structures for movement — become tight and unyielding, it can put strain on the little toe and outside of the foot, rather than on the big toe and inside of the foot, where it belongs. If foot muscles are sufficiently out of balance, the long bones of the foot will end up doing most of the work, rather than the toes. In this severe case, the toes often curl. So if you

have a square foot, you should wear a square shoe. If your foot is wide across the ball, the shoe you buy should match. If your foot or heel is narrow, choose accordingly. Consider a shoe that ties if your arch is so high that the top of your foot rubs the top of the shoe: laces can accommodate this hereditary feature.

Sole: choose a shoe appropriate for the surface on which you walk most often. A soft-soled shoe is preferable for most surfaces — it absorbs some of the shock that a hard floor repels. However, researchers at the Nike Corporation have found evidence that suggests that hard-soled shoes may be more appropriate for standing on hard surfaces. As the body struggles to maintain a standing position, the muscles necessary to keep the body upright constantly shift. The stable pedestal offered by a hard-soled shoe works best for a foot that is constantly shifting in place.

Soft shoes

A new generation of shoes has recently been developed specifically for walking at work, for sport and for leisure. They have in common the factors of a soft sole, a wide toe box to allow for toe spread, a flexible sole, a low heel and materials that allow air to circulate round the entire foot.

High heels

Any heel over 5 cm (2 in) imposes deformity on the body, such as shortened calf muscles, metatarsal damage and problems in the lower back, shoulders and neck. Studies show that high heels require greater expenditure of energy over a distance. That tired feeling at the end of a day can result from the self-imposed handicap of heels.

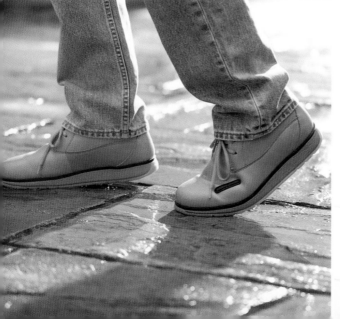

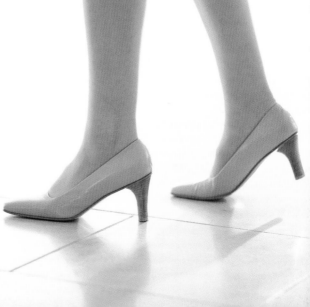

HEALTH PATHWAYS

We call health pathways "Disneyland for the feet" because they take the structures of the feet on a brief holiday away from their regular job. Every day, the foot bears all the weight of the body, adjusting in response to changes in terrain underfoot. A health pathway uses this weight to turn the mundane activity of walking into a unique sensory experience for the feet that reduces stress not only in the foot itself, but throughout the body. By using health pathways, you can lift your arches while lifting your spirits.

Health pathways are walkways, homemade or commercially produced, composed of unusually shaped items. Walking along these pathways on bare feet stimulates previously neglected parts of the feet, thereby breaking up the stress of repetitive actions on the feet and extending to relieve stress throughout the body.

The tradition of health pathways is enjoying a revival in Asia among many people seeking to improve their health. The idea recalls the Japanese legend that Samurai warriors would chop down a piece of bamboo and walk on the rounded surface to promote strength and vigour, an exercise known as *takefumi*. Because the sole is viewed as the body's "second heart" in Japanese tradition, ageing was seen to begin at the feet. The strength of the sole equated with the strength of the soul, or so the idea goes.

Japan's first modern health pathway was created in the 1980s at the Shiseido Cosmetics Factory in Kakegawa, Japan. It comprises a 75-metre (250-foot) walk round an irregular rectangle and features three large types of gravel set within a flat mortar path, the stimulus beginning softly and gradually becoming stronger. There are bridges of small gravel to stimulate the toes, square stones designed to confront hard-to-reach areas with a strong stimulus and large square stones with sharp edges laid flat. Small gravel,

challenging for the bottoms of toes or areas between the toes, is juxtaposed with rounded concrete bars and stones, effective for the arches and designed to replicate the motion of the traditional health exercise of walking on bamboo, *takefumi*.

MAKING YOUR OWN PATHWAY

To replicate the effect at home, incorporate some of the ideas set out on pages 48–49 to create your own health pathway, either indoors or in your garden. Lay a trail of different surface textures to walk over or stand still on. Choose whatever appeals to you, and give yourself the chance to play, trying new items to keep yourself interested and to stimulate your feet in different ways. Choose from the handle of a broom or wooden dowelling; crunchy gravel, pebbles and smooth river rocks; found objects from the beach, woodlands or garden, such as driftwood, a fallen log or a rounded concrete lawn edger; rounded bamboo or a PVC pipe cut in half; a door mat, sand and soothing grass. When using outdoor items, be sure they remain stable — bury them in earth or support them in some other way. Indoors, consider using small, stable objects, or place items in a container or tray. For example, place dried peas in a box or rocks in a sock. For support while static, hold on to the back of a chair. Some people like

Using a health pathway

1 To work statically, stand with hands resting on a chair back for support and place one foot on a broomstick.

2 Slowly shift your body weight onto the stick, rolling it underfoot and using it to massage every part of the sole. Note the different sensations it evokes in different parts of the foot, and any areas of discomfort.

BENEFITS OF PATHWAYS

Boosted overall energy levels

Deep sleep

Feet that feel fully relaxed

A sense of strength in the muscles of the foot, legs, abdomen and lower back

VARIATIONS

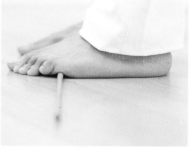

If a broomstick seems too painful, try a less challenging object, such as a dowel stick of lesser diameter.

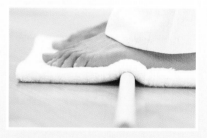

Alternatively, cover the broomstick with a towel before applying pressure to it. After a few sessions you may be able to remove the towel.

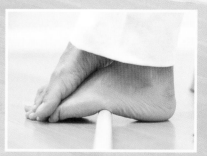

If this is still too powerful, start from a seated position, using one foot on top of the other to exert pressure onto the stick and accustom your foot to the rounded surface. Gradually build up to the full standing position in step 1.

to stand in one place and work with one piece of interesting surface underfoot, while others like to take a hike, walking over a variety of surfaces. The optimal

These exercises give the foot an opportunity to explore shapes that were once part of its everyday experience.

frequency and duration of application should be every day for about 10 minutes, so make sure to choose a variety of experiences you actively enjoy.

STARTING OUT

Health pathways are a form of exercise, so start out gradually. As with any exercise, you should consult a medical practitioner prior to proceeding if you have an existing foot or medical problem, such as osteoporosis,

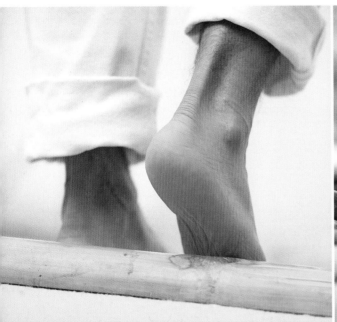

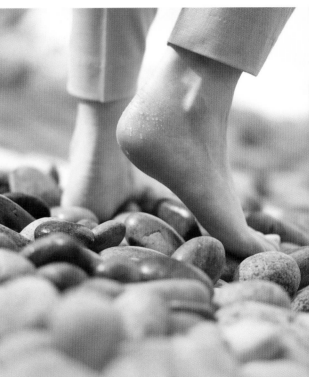

Bare feet on bamboo

Takefumi is the Japanese tradition of walking on bamboo: *take* means "bamboo" and *fumi* "to step upon". Take a length of bamboo cut in half and place it rounded side up on the floor. Stand and place one foot on the bamboo. Slowly shift your body weight onto the surface, noting what you feel and any areas of sensitivity. Your foot should feel pleasantly rather than unpleasantly stressed. Experiment by rocking from side to side, or vary the dimension by working with bamboo (or PVC piping) of different dimensions.

Bare feet on stones

Rocks smoothed by running water can provide a pleasant surface on which to exercise the feet. Experiment by sampling a variety of rocks – you may discover that you have a favourite size and dimension of pebble. You may even find that one rock feels particularly good to one part of the foot, while another stone feels good to another. In addition to applying pressure with a single stone, stand or walk (carefully) in a rocky riverbed to appreciate the invigorating sensation of cool running water.

or any other concerns. Before using a health pathway, remember that any object you step on is a challenge to the foot. Be aware of the effect each texture has on your foot, noting your response and staying within your comfort zone. If you over-challenge your foot, you may make yourself susceptible to injury. If you feel soreness in the foot after walking on a pathway, reduce the challenge by shortening the amount of time you use your health pathway or changing to a smaller

object. If, after attaining positive results with your first pathway, you wish to step up a level, try adapting the pathway to include more challenging objects and textures to walk over or stand on. Examples of these might include stones with the sharper edges laid flat, or a combination of smaller gradations of gravel to really work the bottoms of the toes and the spaces between them and more rounded objects to manipulate the arches.

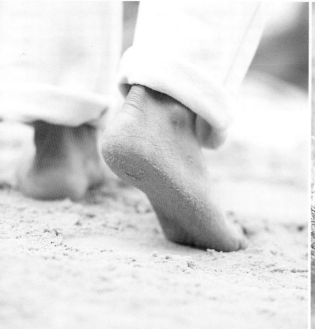

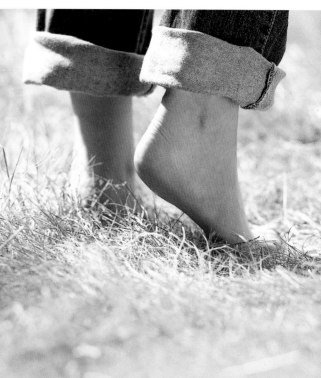

Bare feet on sand

Walking barefoot on sand provides a workout for all the muscles found in the foot and calf. This shifting surface gives under pressure from the foot, making the foot work harder than it would on concrete or other flat, stable surfaces, and push off the ground in a very different way, too. Thus, walking on sand not only provides good physical exercise for the feet, but gives the whole body a workout as well.

Bare feet on grass

Stepping on grass can be cool and refreshing, and the soft and springy sole of the foot appreciates its reciprocating soft springiness. Try walking on grass at different times of day – first thing in the morning when moistened by dew; following a rain shower when the ground is sodden; and at night, when your sense of sight cannot distract from the sensations underfoot. Appreciate grass in different seasons, too, from a crunchy winter frost to springtime grass warmed by the sun.

SELF-HELP TOOLS

Reflexology tools can help pinpoint the locations of stresses in your feet, hands and body. They then go one step further to break up or interrupt those stresses. Consider how much time and money you have available. If your financial resources are limited, you can create your own self-help device using household items, such as golf balls. If your time comes at a premium, you can even use your self-help tool discreetly while working at your desk or standing in a queue.

LEARNING TIP

Remember that tools are only for self-help and never for application of pressure on someone else. Be aware of your response to the pressure exerted by the hard surface of tools such as foot rollers or golf balls. Choose a level of pressure according to your preference and level of comfort.

Hand and foot self-help tools come in a variety of shapes and sizes. Shown here are some cylindrical foot rollers and a spherical roller for use on either the hands or the feet.

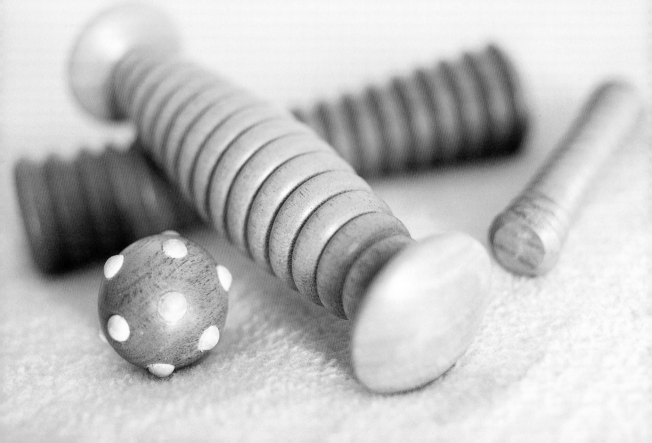

Self-help tools for the feet

Cylindrical objects work best when rolled under the foot. In addition to commercially available products, you can use objects found round the house, including rolling pins, soft-drink bottles or the rung of a chair. A golf ball is an ideal self-help tool because of its appropriate size and shape.

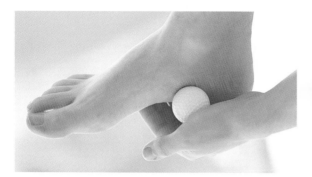

Cup the golf ball in the palm of your hand, trapping it against your foot. Rest your fingers on the outside edge of your foot. Roll the golf ball through the area.

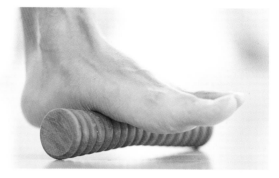

Place your foot on the roller. Roll your foot along the roller, angling the foot to target different reflex areas. You may increase the pressure by crossing your legs.

Self-help tools for the hands

Using hand tools usually requires little effort, and they are often more discreet and easier to use than foot tools. Golf balls or even small, round dog toys are convenient items for application of pressure.

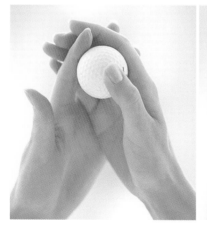

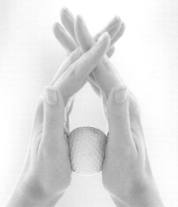

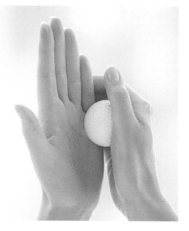

Target the fingers and thumb by trapping the digit to be worked between the golf ball and the fingers of your other hand. Roll the ball along the entire digit.

Work reflex areas in the heels of the hands by lacing the fingers together. Place the ball between the heels of the hands and roll the ball throughout the area.

To pinpoint an area, cup the golf ball in one hand, holding it in place by resting the fingers of your other hand on top. Roll the golf ball throughout the area.

RELAXATION EXERCISES

For the feet

A footstep is made possible by the actions of and interactions between muscles, tendons and ligaments, but these areas seldom experience their full range of movement during the routine activities of a normal day. To break up your routine and strengthen the foot's structures, try the following exercises.

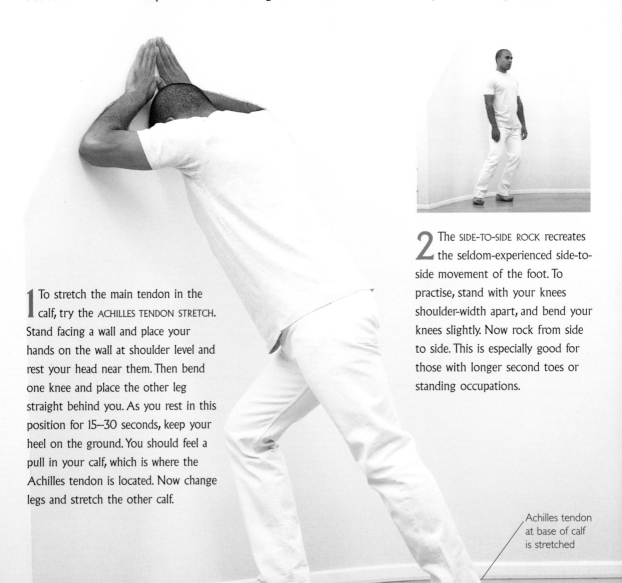

1 To stretch the main tendon in the calf, try the ACHILLES TENDON STRETCH. Stand facing a wall and place your hands on the wall at shoulder level and rest your head near them. Then bend one knee and place the other leg straight behind you. As you rest in this position for 15–30 seconds, keep your heel on the ground. You should feel a pull in your calf, which is where the Achilles tendon is located. Now change legs and stretch the other calf.

2 The SIDE-TO-SIDE ROCK recreates the seldom-experienced side-to-side movement of the foot. To practise, stand with your knees shoulder-width apart, and bend your knees slightly. Now rock from side to side. This is especially good for those with longer second toes or standing occupations.

Achilles tendon at base of calf is stretched

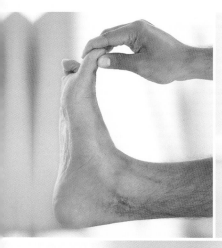
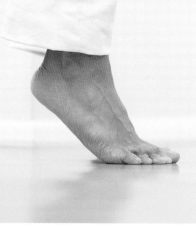
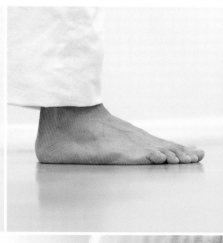

3 TOE STRETCHES can be done while seated. With your foot resting on your knee, grasp your big toe, pulling it gently and slowly to stretch the muscles on the bottom of the foot. Repeat on all toes of both feet.

4 TOE RAISES strengthen the muscles in the bottoms of the feet and the calf. While standing, grasp the back of a chair to balance yourself. Rise onto the balls of the feet, pause, then lower. Repeat several times.

5 While standing or sitting, practise the TOE PRESS by pressing down on the floor with the toes to strengthen the muscles of the toes. Try to imagine pushing your toes down completely flat on the floor.

6 The ANKLE ROTATION loosens and stretches foot muscles, and improves circulation to the ankles. First circle the foot in a clockwise direction several times, then repeat the circle in an anti-clockwise direction several times. As you draw a full circle in the air with your big toe, the foot should move through all four directional movements. Now repeat on the other foot.

For the hands

The habitual patterns followed by the hands during the day are limited and this can lead to strain and injury. The goal of these exercises is to provide the hands with a fuller range of movement than they normally experience in order to break up these stress patterns.

For those who regularly perform a repetitive task such as typing, steps 3–6, known as the directional movements of the hand, are particularly useful.

1 To try the FINGER-PULL, wrap one hand round the index finger of the other hand, and pull gently and slowly outwards. Hold for several seconds. Repeat on each digit, including the thumb. To test the effect of this technique, open and close your fingers. The hand you've just worked should feel more relaxed than the other. Repeat on the other hand.

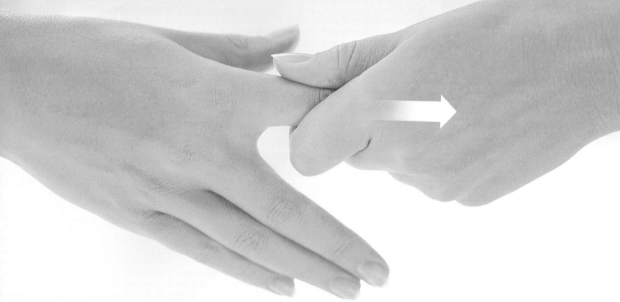

2 Next, loosen up your palms with the PALM-MOVER. Position your hand so that your other fingers now rest on the top of your other hand, while your thumb sits on the surface of the palm. Press down with your fingers while pushing up with your thumb. The movement created is similar to that of wringing your hands. Do this several times and then repeat on the other hand.

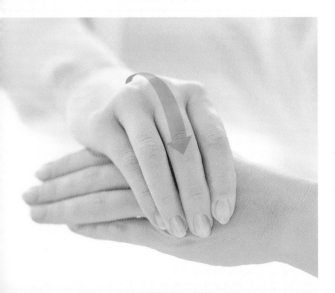

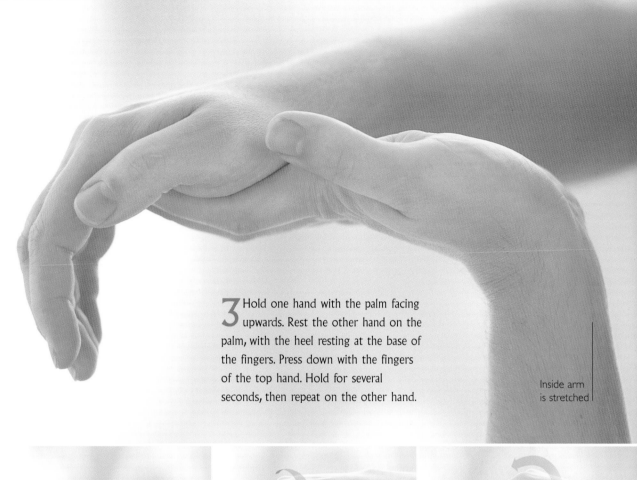

3 Hold one hand with the palm facing upwards. Rest the other hand on the palm, with the heel resting at the base of the fingers. Press down with the fingers of the top hand. Hold for several seconds, then repeat on the other hand.

Inside arm is stretched

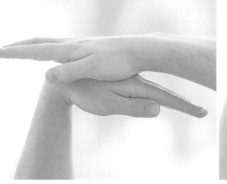

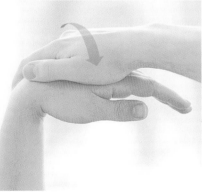

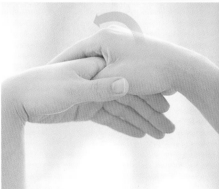

4 Next, rest one hand on top of the other. Press down with the heel of the hand for a few seconds before applying the same exercise on the other hand.

5 Now rest one hand on top of the other. Wrap your fingers round the outside of the hand. Press down with the heel of the top hand, holding the position briefly. Now repeat on your other hand.

6 Finally, with one hand on top of the other, wrap your fingers round the inside of the hand, pressing down with the fingers of the top hand. Hold momentarily and repeat on the other hand.

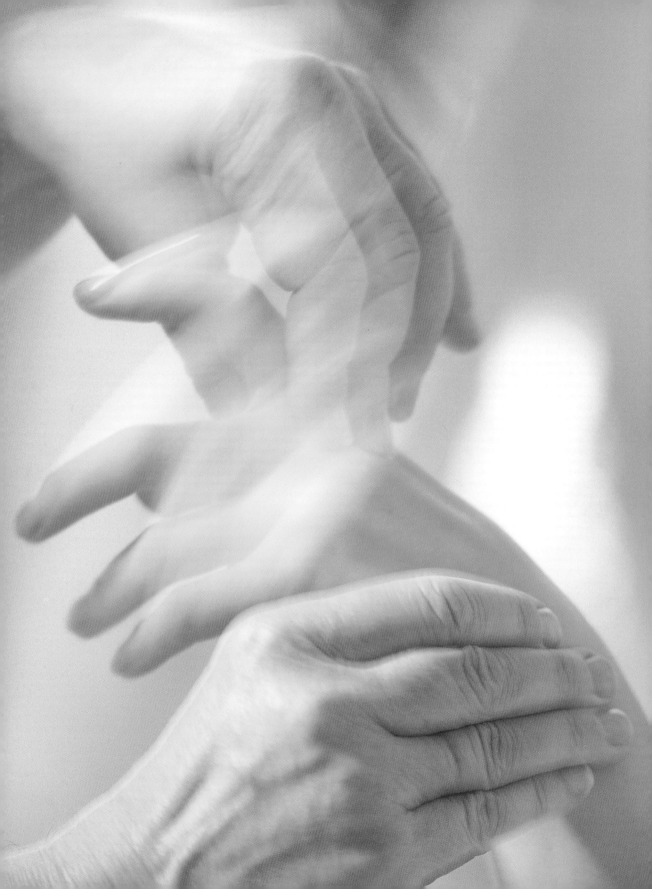

GIVING A REFLEXOLOGY SESSION

This chapter guides you, step by step, through a complete hand and foot reflexology sequence. "Desserts" applied at the beginning and end of each "step" aim to promote a sense of relaxation. There's also a handy self-help section, which shows you how to give yourself a discreet workout, and offers advice on the needs of babies and children, pregnant women and the elderly. Following these sequences regularly can help restore your body to full health.

PREPARING FOR A REFLEXOLOGY SESSION

As you prepare to give a reflexology workout, your goal should be to create a relaxing interchange between yourself and a friend or relative. You want to have the maximum effect with the minimum amount of effort. This includes creating a comfortable setting for yourself and the other individual, paying attention to the effect of your work, and even selecting an appropriate time.

In creating your ideal setting for a reflexology session, consider what is available to you and what you find comfortable. Place your arms next to your body. Now raise your hands so that your elbows are bent at a 90° angle. This is an optimal position for your working hands. The feet or hands on which you are working should be placed in a position comfortably reached by your working hands.

For a session with a professional reflexologist, the individual is seated in a recliner or other chair that raises the feet into position. The reflexologist sits in a low chair facing the reclining chair. You may prefer a more informal setting, such as sitting on a sofa facing each other. Whatever your working arrangement, be in a position to watch the individual's face for his or her reaction to your work. Be careful that your back is supported and that your work doesn't cause aching or stress to your own body. (Once you've finished your work, think about how you feel. Are your hands stressed and is your back tired?)

OPTIMUM POSITIONING

When working on the hands, sitting side by side with the individual works well, as long as you ensure that you can still see his or her face. Change sides to work on the other hand. When working with a child, you may choose to sit on the side of the bed for a quiet few minutes at bedtime and give a brief foot workout then.

Sitting with the individual's face in your view allows you to gauge his or her reactions to your work. Falling asleep and smiles are good. Frowns and pulling the foot away are bad. You want to apply reflexology technique within the individual's comfort zone. There's an old saying in reflexology: it hurts good. (Yes, people do say this.) The counterpart is: it hurts bad. Keep an eye on the individual's face to see what techniques are favoured and which reflex areas are sensitive. Also, be aware of how much pressure you are using. A child, a small individual, the elderly, or anyone with thin feet will require less pressure than a large man, for example.

ACCESSORIES AND ENVIRONMENT

Take time to assemble a few accessories. A few cushions are handy to raise the level of the foot or to provide cushioning on which the hand or foot will rest as you work. A coverlet or light blanket is helpful – you may be warm because you are working, but the other person is resting and may become chilled. A box of tissues is convenient for the occasional running nose.

Consider the environment. What would you like yourself? If your goal is to create the ultimate relaxing moment or a quiet time for conversation, you may want to limit distractions such as a ringing telephone, other people in the room, the television, bright lighting, even what is in the sightline of the individual. Communicate to find out what your mutual ideal

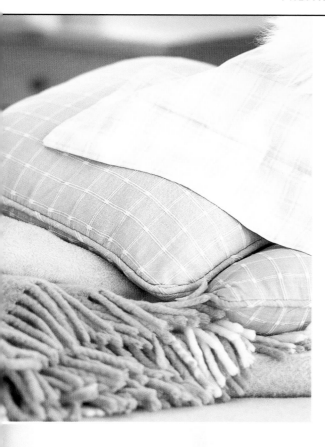

environment would be. For your own part, you may actually appreciate as few distractions as possible, especially as you learn.

A further element of preparation involves your fingernails. Nails should not be too long or too short. If too long they will make contact with the receiver's foot or hand and detract from relaxation. If you see fingernail marks on the foot or hand, consider trimming your nails. The optimal length for fingernails is when your fingertips, rather than your fingernails, are visible as you look at the tops of your hands. If your nails are cut too short, as far back as the quick, it could prove to be uncomfortable as the nail pulls away from the skin underneath.

The techniques described in this book do not involve cream, oil or lotion. Like running in wet sand, these emollients can create over-work for your thumbs and damage them. Likewise the individual you are working with should have clean feet, free of emollients.

BEGINNING THE SESSION

Always begin your work with a series of desserts (*see page 68*). Desserts play an important part in the workout. The workout follows a specific pattern, enabling you to work through the entire foot or hand. As you work through each section of the foot or hand, apply a series of desserts before going on to the next section. As you finish your work, apply a further series of desserts.

How long should technique be applied to any individual reflex area? The answer to this question is tailored to the individual with whom you are working. Infants, children and the elderly generally require a light touch: less pressure and less time are the watchwords as it is possible to overwork a reflex area. If the individual reports that the area feels bruised, it has been over-worked. Avoid the area until sensitivity diminishes and work it less when your reflexology work begins again.

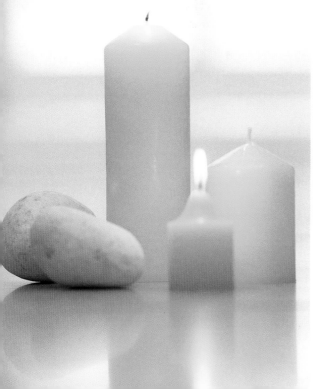

Candles can help to create a relaxing atmosphere for a reflexology session, while cushions and blankets are useful for keeping the receiver warm and comfortable while his or her feet or hands are being worked.

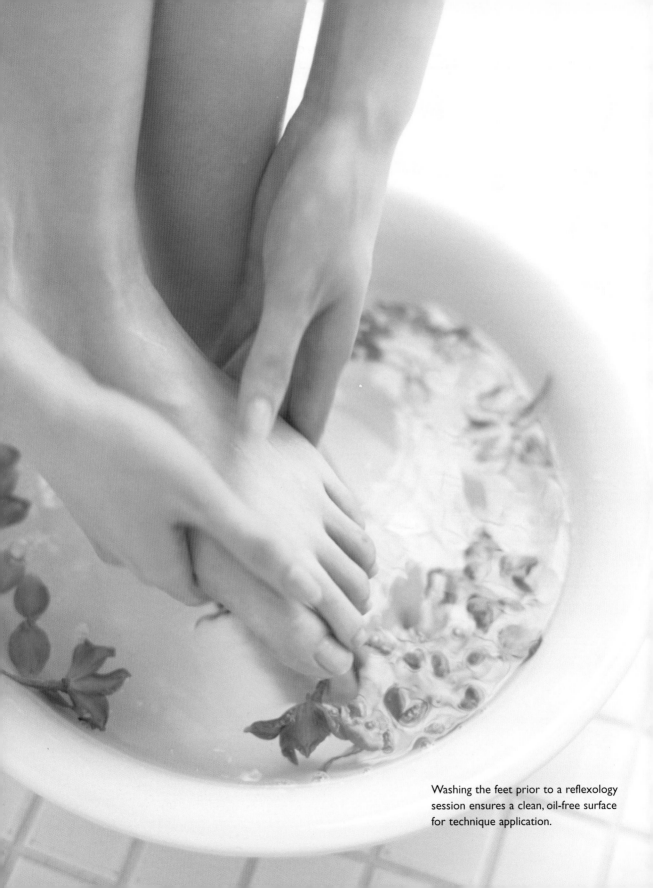

Washing the feet prior to a reflexology session ensures a clean, oil-free surface for technique application.

A professional reflexologist will spend anywhere from 30 minutes to an hour providing a workout. At the beginning of your work with reflexology, you will find that your hands and thumb may tire. Half an hour may be too much. If so, there are several strategies for avoiding fatigue (*see box below*).

TREATING DISORDERS

After you've worked through the foot, it's time to consider areas of emphasis. These are areas that need extra attention. To choose such areas, consider your goals. Is there a specific health problem of concern? If so, turn to chapter 5, Reflexology to Treat Disorders, and find your health concern. Note the reflex areas listed and apply technique to them. Or consult the reflexology charts (*see pages 16–23*). Apply a series of desserts again, after working any specific areas.

Now move on to the other foot, where you'll repeat the above. When you've finished your work with the second foot, it's time for a closing technique, such as a gentle breathing hold (*see above right*).

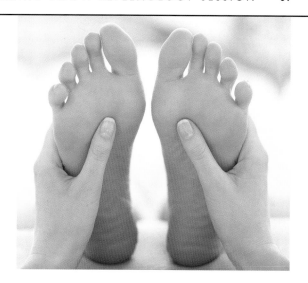

End a session by placing your thumbs in the solar plexus reflex areas of each foot, pressing slightly and asking the receiver to take three slow, deep breaths with you.

TIPS FOR AVOIDING TIREDNESS

TIME: Give yourself time to learn – just as with acquiring any skill, practice and time are needed.

POSITION: Make sure you have a comfortable working position that does not put unnecessary stresses and strains on your body.

TECHNIQUE: Review your technique application – done properly, your hands should not tire too easily.

STRENGTH: Practise self-help reflexology (see *pages 124–29*) to help build your strength.

DESSERTS: Take a tip from the professionals and break up your work with "desserts" (see *pages 68–73*), since these provide a chance for your working thumb or finger to have a rest.

CHANGE HANDS: Swap working hands regularly – if one thumb tires, adapt and apply technique with your other thumb.

KEY TO TECHNIQUE SYMBOLS

Finger-walking	
Thumb-walking	
Hook & back-up	
Rolling	
Pressure	
Traction, pulling, pushing, or side-to-side	
Rotation or rotation on a point	
Twist	
Sole-mover or palm-rocker	

TECHNIQUES

There are four basic techniques used in reflexology. Their purpose is to apply pressure over a broad area, or to pinpoint a more specific one. As with any skill, it takes time to build ability, so it is a good idea to practise them on your forearm or hand. If your thumb or finger becomes tired while you're learning, rest, change hands or apply desserts (*see pages 68–73 and 98–101*) instead.

Thumb-walking

The goal of the thumb-walking technique is to apply a constant, steady pressure to the surface of the foot or hand. This basic reflexology technique will require some practice. Be patient. Give yourself some time to acquire this valuable skill. It will enable you to help yourself and others to reach health goals.

LEARNING TIP

Thumb-walking is made easier by the use of the proper angle of the thumb. Lay your hands down on a table or flat surface. Note how the thumb rests on the table. The outside edge now making contact with the table is the part of the thumb that should make contact with the surface to be worked. By using this area of the thumb, you take best advantage of the leverage available from the four fingers.

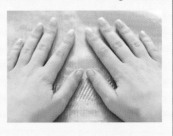

Practising the technique

The basis for the thumb-walking technique is the bending and unbending of the first joint of the thumb. The goal is to take small "bites" to create a feeling of constant, steady pressure.

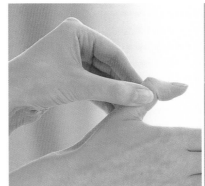

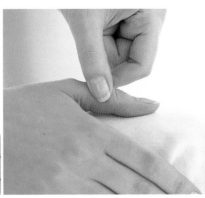

1 First practise the thumb action by holding the thumb below the first joint to prevent movement of the second joint. Bend and unbend the first joint several times.

2 Continue holding on to your thumb. Place the outside edge of the thumb on your leg. Bend and unbend it several times, rocking it a little from the thumb tip to the lower edge of the nail.

Applying the technique

To thumb-walk on the foot or hand, first create a smooth, even surface for your thumb's work. This can be achieved by using the hand not occupied with thumb-walking as the holding hand.

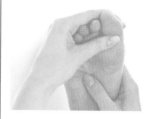
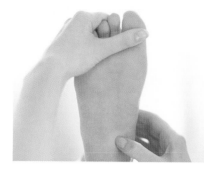

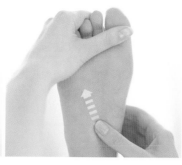

1 With the holding hand, stretch the sole of the foot. Rest your working thumb on the sole and your fingers on the top of the foot. Drop your wrist to create leverage, which exerts pressure with the thumb.

2 Bend and unbend the thumb's first joint, moving it forwards a little bit at a time. When your working hand feels stretched, reposition it and continue "walking" it forwards.

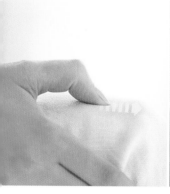

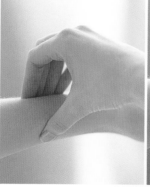

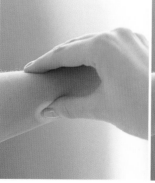

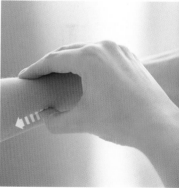

3 Remove the holding hand from your thumb. Walk the thumb forwards. Bending and unbending are the sole means by which you move forwards. Do not push the thumb forwards.

4 To practise using leverage, place the fingers and thumb of your right hand on your forearm as shown. Working together, these create the leverage needed to generate pressure.

5 Lower your wrist so that the thumb exerts pressure on your arm. This pressure is directed through the thumb, but actually results from the actions of the fingers, hand and forearm.

6 Now bend and unbend your thumb, taking a little step forwards with each "unbend". Continue practising on your forearm until you feel a constant, steady pressure.

Finger-walking

The finger-walking technique is used to work comfortably on the top and sides of the foot or hand. Many of the principles of thumb-walking apply (*see page 62*). This technique is based on the same principle as thumb-walking: the bending and unbending of the first joint of the digit.

Practising the technique

The top of the hand is a good practice ground for finger-walking, which is very similar to thumb-walking. The walking motion is created by a slight rocking back and forth from the fingertip to the lower edge of the fingernail, as the finger bends and unbends.

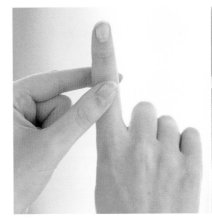

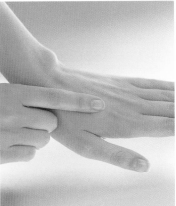

1 Hold the index finger below the first knuckle to help isolate the joint used in the technique (*see above*). Practise bending and unbending the first joint of the finger.

2 Once you have become familiar with the bending and unbending action required, place your index finger on top of your other hand.

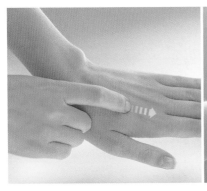

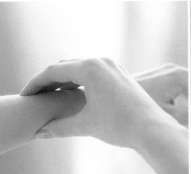

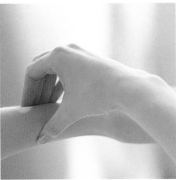

3 Try bending and unbending the index finger from the first joint as its tip rests on top of the hand. Rock the fingertip to the lower edge of the fingernail and back. Repeat several times.

4 To create leverage using the finger-walking technique, use the thumb in opposition to the fingers. Practise this by placing the four fingers on the forearm with the thumb underneath (*see above*).

5 Raise the wrist, holding on with the thumb and pressing the fingers into the forearm. Note the increased pressure now exerted by the finger. Maintaining this position, "walk" the index finger forwards.

Applying the technique

As with thumb-walking, finger-walking on the foot requires a stationary work surface. You can use your holding hand to steady the foot or hand.

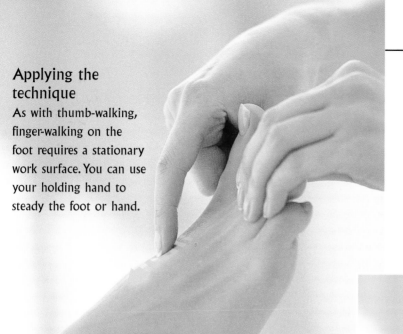

1 The holding hand steadies the foot in an upright position by holding the toes. Rest your index finger on top of the foot and the thumb on the bottom.

2 With the working hand, use the index finger to finger walk down the top of the foot towards the middle.

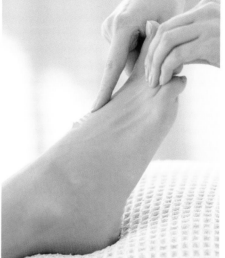

LEARNING TIP

Frequently the finger will "learn" the finger-walking technique on its own, seemingly from one's ability to apply thumb-walking. As with thumb-walking, the finger always moves in a forwards direction, never backwards or sideways.

COMMON MISTAKES

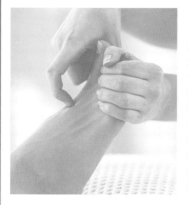

Problems can occur. Usually they involve difficulty in bending the first joint. Try to avoid the following: moving your hand rather than the first joint of the finger; digging the fingernail into the skin; allowing the walking finger to draw back rather than exerting a forwards pressure; and rolling the walking finger from side-to-side. If you encounter any of these difficulties, review your technique by closely re-reading the instructions opposite.

Rotating on a point

As implied by the name, the object of this technique is to pinpoint a reflex area with the middle finger of one hand and then rotate the ankle or wrist. As the joint turns, the middle finger of the working hand stays stationary. This contact between the rotating foot and the static finger creates an "on/off" pressure.

<table>
<tr><td>

LEARNING TIP

Do not grasp the foot round the toes. Also, the pinpointed area on the inside of the ankle is a sensitive area. Rather than pressing with your fingers, allow the turning of the ankle to create pressure.

</td></tr>
</table>

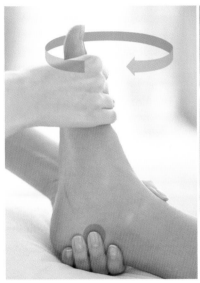

1 With the holding hand, cup the heel so that the thumb rests round the ankle. Allow the middle finger to rest on the inside of the ankle. With the other hand, hold the ball of the foot and rotate the foot clockwise, turning the foot in a complete 360° circle. Maintain a constant pressure of movement as you turn the foot, and notice that an on/off pressure is created by the static middle finger of your holding hand. Rotate in a clockwise direction several times.

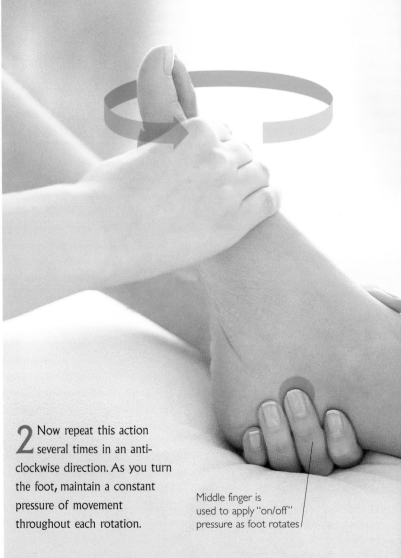

2 Now repeat this action several times in an anti-clockwise direction. As you turn the foot, maintain a constant pressure of movement throughout each rotation.

Middle finger is used to apply "on/off" pressure as foot rotates

Hook & back-up

The hook and back-up technique is used to work a specific point, rather than to cover a large area. It is a relatively stationary technique, with only small movements of the working thumb involved.

Practising the technique

As with all techniques, leverage is extremely important in working with deeper points. Just as in the case of thumb-walking, leverage is provided by the fingers and the position of the wrist.

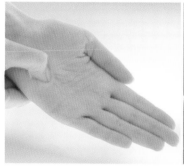

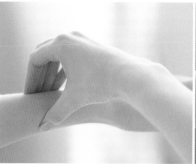

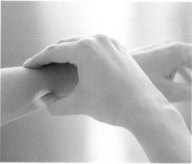

1 Rest your working thumb on the palm of the other hand, placing your fingers on top. Bend the thumb's first joint, resting on the edge of the thumb. Now pull back with the thumb to exert pressure.

2 To practise using leverage, place the four fingers and the thumb of the working hand on the forearm (*see above*).

3 Lower the wrist of the working hand, causing the thumb to exert increased pressure on the arm. With the wrist lowered, hook in with the thumb and pull back.

Applying the technique

The holding hand needs to keep the area stationary as this technique is applied.

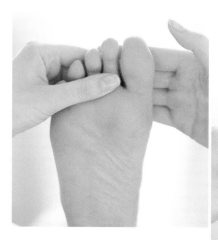

1 Support and protect the area to be worked with holding hand. The hand wraps round the area while the thumb and fingers hold it in place. Place the fingers of the working hand over those of the holding hand (*see right*).

2 Place the working thumb in the centre of the area to be worked. Hook and back-up, using the edge of the thumb.

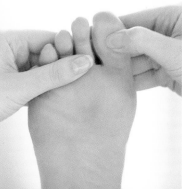

FOOT DESSERTS

A "dessert" technique is something almost everyone likes. These desserts are techniques designed to relax the foot. They provide a beginning, an end, a transition between techniques and a soothing touch when sensitivity is a problem. In helping to relax the foot, they make your work as a reflexologist easier, because a relaxed person is more receptive to technique application.

> ## LEARNING TIP
>
> This technique is most effective when applied rhythmically and rapidly. Keep your hands at the ball of the foot. Rest them lightly but firmly on the foot. Do not press too hard, since this will restrict the foot's movement. As you practise, you will become more adept at a quicker pace, with the strength to apply it for longer periods of time.

Side-to-side

This technique uses a side-to-side motion to relax the foot. In this dessert, the foot is turned from side-to-side and in and out. Since the foot is usually restricted to the up-and-down movement of footsteps during the course of a day, this technique provides a particularly enjoyable variation.

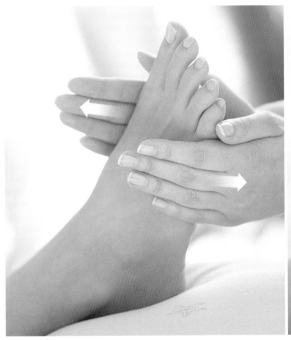

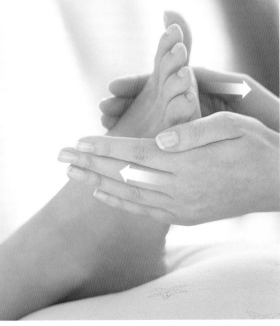

1 Rest the hands on the sides of the foot. With the right hand, move the side of the foot away from you, while moving the other side towards you with your left hand.

2 Now move the right hand back towards you, pulling that side of the foot round, while pushing the other side of the foot away from you with the left hand. Alternate the actions of the hands, moving the sides of the foot quickly back and forth.

Spinal twist

This dessert is so named because it provides relaxation for the spinal reflex area along the inside of the foot. It is most comfortable if all digits make firm contact with the foot.

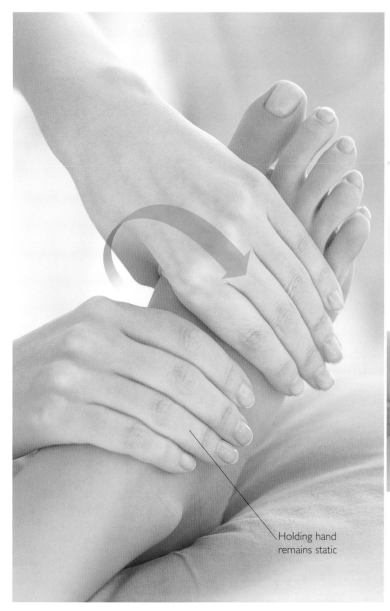

Holding hand remains static

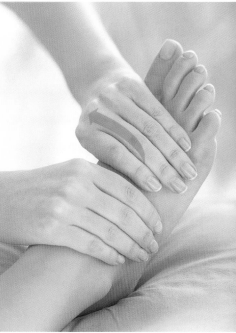

1 Grasp the inside of the foot with both hands, the thumbs resting on the sole of the foot. With the hand closest to the toes, turn the foot. The other hand remains stationary.

2 Now move the same hand in the opposite direction, again keeping the hand nearest the ankle static. Repeat, twisting the foot gently from side to side several times. Reposition the hands, moving them both towards the ankle slightly, and repeat the whole movement several times again.

Lung press

This dessert is so named because it provides relaxation to the lung reflex area in the ball of the foot. The art in this dessert lies in the smooth, wave-like motion created by co-ordinating the movements of the two hands. Think of the ebb and flow of a wave. One hand pushes and the other hand responds with a gentle squeeze.

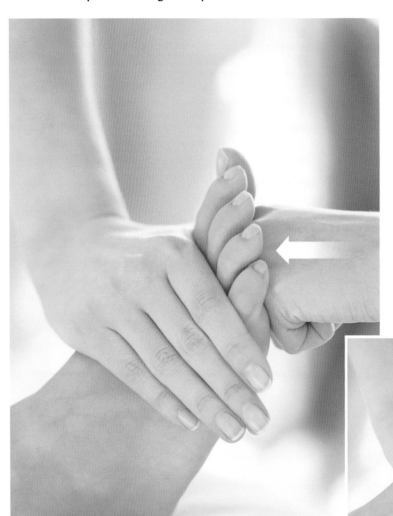

1 Make a fist with the left hand. Rest the flat of the fist against the ball of the foot. Grasp the top of the foot with the right hand. Push with the fist.

2 Now squeeze gently with the right hand. Develop a rhythmic push/squeeze pattern as you repeat the actions several times.

Sole-mover

The goal of this technique is to create movement in the bones that make up the ball of the foot. It provides relaxation for the lung, chest, upper back and diaphragm reflex areas – all common areas for stress.

1 Grasp the ball of the foot below the big toe and second toe. Rest your finger and thumb tips on the knobby heads of the bones in the ball of the foot. Move the foot away from you with the right hand and towards you with the left hand.

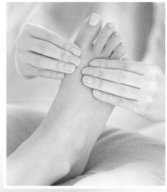

Rest your fingertips on the top side of the foot, with the tips of your thumbs on the underside.

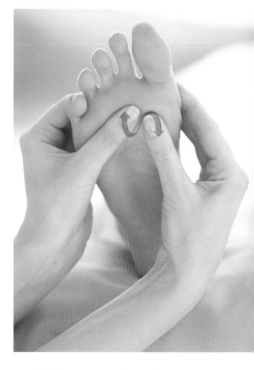

2 Now reverse the motions, moving the foot towards you with the right hand and away from you with the left. Repeat this pattern several times, establishing a rhythm. Go on to the ball of the foot below the second and third toes and apply this technique. Do the same with the third and fourth, and then the fourth and fifth toes.

Ankle rotation

This dessert is also an exercise. By turning the foot in a complete 360° circle, you are exercising and relaxing the four major muscle groups that control the movements of the foot. It also helps ease fluid retention round the ankles.

Toe rotation

This dessert both gently relaxes the toes and strengthens them at the same time as it works their muscles fully.

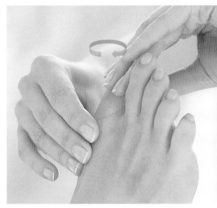

1 Keep the top of the foot steady with the holding hand. Grasp the big toe with the other hand. Rotate the toe slowly and evenly in a 360° clockwise circle several times.

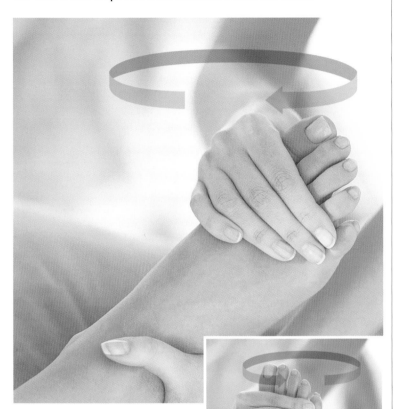

1 Grasp the ankle with your holding hand. Using your other hand, hold the ball of the foot and rotate the toes in a clockwise direction to make a 360° circle. Repeat several times.

LEARNING TIP

Rest the thumb of the holding hand below the ankle bone. Pull the foot towards you with the holding hand, and then turn it with the other hand.

2 Now move the foot in an anti-clockwise direction. Repeat several times.

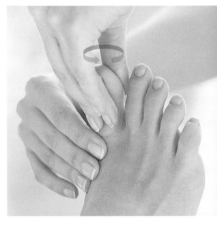

2 Now rotate the toe in an anti-clockwise direction. Use firm, even pressure with the working fingers and a slight upwards pull. Apply to each of the toes.

Traction

This is a good technique for overall relaxation of the foot. It counteracts the continual compression of the foot that occurs with each footstep.

1 Grasp the foot as shown (*see right*). Pull the foot towards you, gently and gradually. Hold for 10–15 seconds. Release.

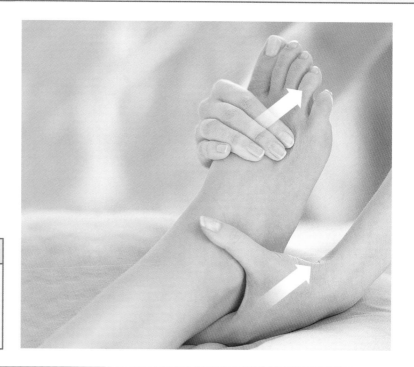

LEARNING TIP

As you move the ball of the foot towards you with the working hand, pull simultaneously at the ankle with the holding hand.

Mid-foot mover

The joint across the centre of the foot is often compressed from footwear and standing for long periods of time. The net result is stress on the foot in general, as well as on the reflex areas of the mid-foot. The mid-foot mover breaks up the stress experienced by the middle of the foot.

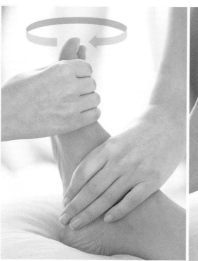

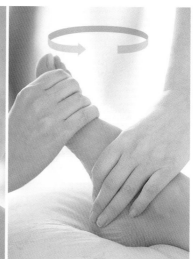

LEARNING TIP

As you move the foot, work against the holding hand. As a variation, try bridging the ankle rather than the centre of the foot.

1 Bridge your holding hand over the centre of the foot, keeping it static. Grasp the ball of the foot with the other hand and move the ball of the foot 360° in a clockwise direction. Repeat several times.

2 Now turn the foot in an anti-clockwise direction. Repeat several times.

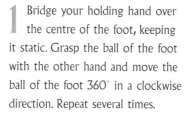

STEP 1

Working the underside of the toes

Many of the reflex areas in this sequence correspond to parts of the anatomy that are responsible for directing many of the body's activities. Some of these areas, like the head and brain, gather information about the outside world. Working the reflex areas in this sequence stimulates and enhances the functions of these organs. First, examine the foot for any areas that should be avoided, and then start with the desserts below to relax the foot.

DESSERTS   Side-to-side (p. 68) • Spinal twist (p. 69)
Lung press (p. 70) • Toe rotation (p. 72)

AREAS WORKED

PITUITARY GLAND: This helps regulate endocrine activity such as growth and metabolism.

NECK: Highly prone to tension, it may respond well to reflexology.

THYROID & PARATHYROID GLANDS: Help to regulate energy levels, metabolism, growth and blood calcium levels: pressure is applied to these reflex areas to enhance the functions of these glands.

HEAD & BRAIN: Control and co-ordinate all activity in the body, so a key part of a reflexology session.

SINUSES: Reflexology work aims to keep these air-filled cavities clear.

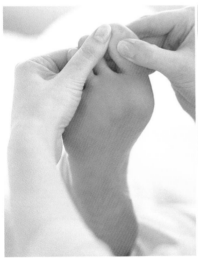 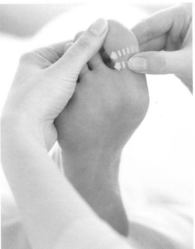 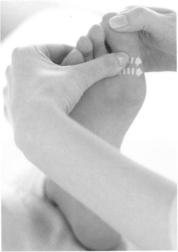

1 Hold the big toe stationary with your left hand. Rest your right thumb just beyond the PITUITARY GLAND reflex area. Hook in with the thumb and pull back across the reflex area. Repeat.

2 Next, place your right thumb on the NECK, THYROID GLAND and PARATHYROID GLAND reflex areas. Walk across the stem of the toe using the thumb-walking technique. Make at least two passes, one high and one low.

3 Change hands and walk across the stem of the toes from the other direction. Make both low and high passes. Repeat several times.

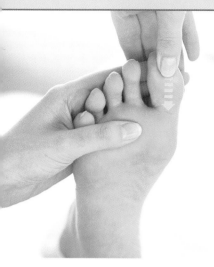

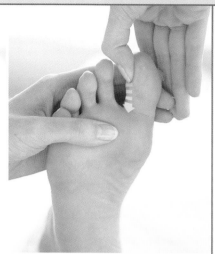

FOOT ORIENTATION

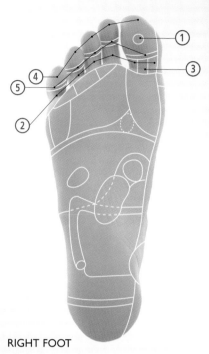

4 To work the HEAD and BRAIN, SINUS and NECK reflex areas, first support the toes with your left hand. Now thumb-walk, starting at the top centre of the big toe.

5 Reposition your right thumb and walk down the side of the big toe.

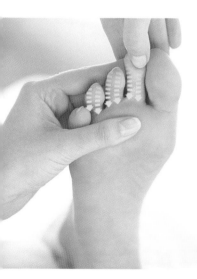

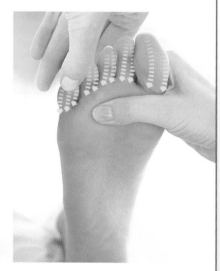

6 Next, reposition your left hand to support the second toe. Walk down the centre and side of this toe. Repeat the pattern on the third and fourth toes.

7 Repeat on the little toe, then change hands. Use the right hand to support each toe and walk the left thumb down the centre and the other side of each toe.

DESSERTS   Side-to-side (p. 68) • Lung press (p. 70) • Toe rotation (p. 72)

RIGHT FOOT

The area representing the PITUITARY GLAND lies in the centre of the big toe on both right and left feet ①. The toes are all mapped to mirror the body, with the NECK reflex areas lying in the section from the base of the toe to the first joint ②. On each foot this section of toe represents a portion of the neck, but on the big toes this section also overlaps with the THYROID and PARATHYROID GLAND areas ③.

The area filling the space from the first joint to the tip of each toe corresponds to the HEAD and BRAIN reflex areas ④, with those for the SINUSES ⑤ lying just behind each joint.

The right and left feet mirror each other identically for these reflex areas, with those on the right foot corresponding to the right half of the body and those on the left relating to the left half of the body.

STEP 2
Working the base of the toes

The reflex areas discussed in this sequence represent a range of body areas, from the eyes, the ears and the inner ears to the tops of the shoulders. Work these areas on the foot to enhance the functioning of corresponding parts of the body. This sequence is helpful if you want to ease tension and pain in the tops of the shoulders. Work the area on the right foot for pain in the right shoulder and that on the left foot for pain in the left shoulder.

AREAS WORKED

EYES: Reflexology may help soothe sore eyes.

INNER EARS: These organs regulate our sense of balance.

EARS: The application of reflexology techniques may help ease an earache or tinnitus.

TOPS OF THE SHOULDERS: This muscular region, which is inclined to store tension, may benefit from reflexology sessions.

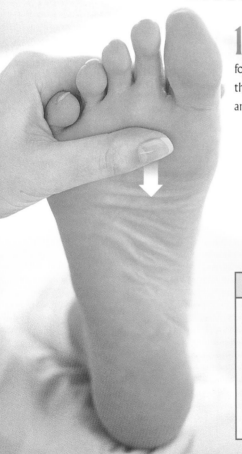

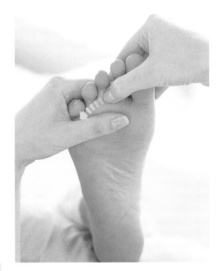

1 Wrap your left hand round the ball of the foot and pull down with the thumb to make the reflex areas more accessible.

LEARNING TIP

Do not squeeze the foot with the holding hand, because that would obscure the surface area of those reflexes. Do not hold the toes back, either, for that would tighten the skin, making it even harder to work the area.

2 Beginning with the EYE reflex area, walk the thumb of your right hand along the top of the ridge. Then thumb-walk along the INNER EAR and EAR reflex areas, along with the reflex area for the TOPS OF THE SHOULDERS, which lies behind the other reflex areas.

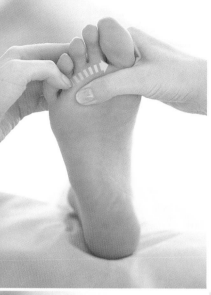

3 Change hands and walk back across the ridge with your left thumb, starting with the EAR reflex area. Walking from both directions ensures that all the reflex areas are thoroughly worked.

FOOT ORIENTATION

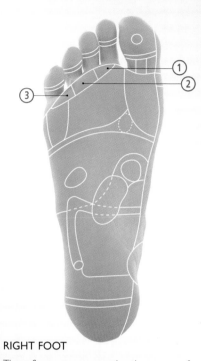

RIGHT FOOT

The reflex areas representing the organs of sight, hearing and balance lie close together, in the part of the foot where the base of the toes meet the sole. The right and left feet mirror each other for these reflex areas, with those on the right foot corresponding to the right half of the body and those on the left relating to the left half of the body.

The EYE reflex area sits just below the space between the second and third toes ①. The INNER EAR reflex area is beneath the space between the third and fourth toes ②, and that of the EAR under the space between the fourth and fifth ③. The reflex area for the TOPS OF THE SHOULDERS lies behind the reflex areas, spanning the entire base of the toes.

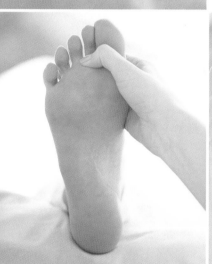

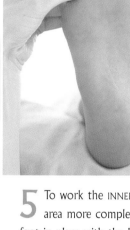

4 To work the EYE reflex area more thoroughly, hold the foot in place with the right hand. Rest the tip of your right thumb and that of your right index finger between the second and third toes, then pinch gently several times.

5 To work the INNER EAR reflex area more completely, hold the foot in place with the left hand. Rest the tip of the thumb and the tip of the index finger between the third and fourth toes, and pinch gently several times. Move on to the EAR reflex area between the fourth and fifth toes and repeat the sequence.

DESSERTS   Side-to-side (p. 68) • Lung press (p. 70) • Sole-mover (p. 71)

STEP 3

Working the ball of the foot

Some of the reflex areas worked in this sequence correspond to the lungs and many other parts of the body involved in breathing and the transport of oxygen round the body. The other reflex areas found in this part of the foot represent sections of the upper body, such as the upper back and the shoulder. You should work these reflex areas to enhance functioning and to relieve tension in these areas of the body.

AREAS WORKED
DIAPHRAGM & SOLAR PLEXUS: Reflexology aims to enhance the performance of this muscle and nerve network, which is involved in respiration and other involuntary body functions.
HEART: This pumps oxygenated blood throughout the body.
CHEST & LUNGS: Apply reflexology to these reflex areas to help keep the chest and lungs open.
UPPER BACK & SHOULDERS: Working these reflex areas may ease tension in the upper torso and the shoulders.

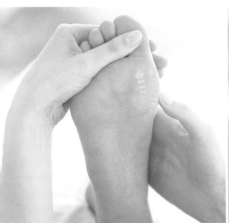 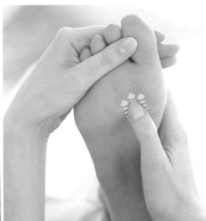 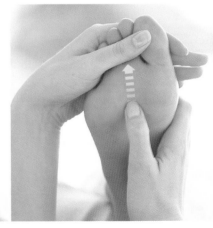

1 Hold the toes back with your left hand. Beginning at the DIAPHRAGM reflex area, use the thumb of the right hand to walk up through the HEART and CHEST reflex areas. Make several passes through this broad area.

2 Move your thumb back to the SOLAR PLEXUS reflex area. Using the same technique as before, make several passes through this small area.

3 Move your thumb to another segment of the DIAPHRAGM reflex area. Thumb-walk up through the LUNG, CHEST and UPPER BACK reflex areas. Make several passes through these areas on the ball of the foot and up between the second and third toes.

FOOT ORIENTATION

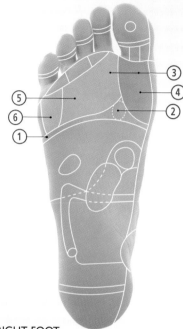

RIGHT FOOT

The reflex area relating to the DIAPHRAGM runs along the length of the horizontal crease below the ball of the foot ①. Within it lies the small SOLAR PLEXUS reflex area ②.

The broad reflex area corresponding to the CHEST and UPPER BACK spans much of the ball of the foot above the diaphragm area ③. It overlaps both the HEART reflex area ④ and the LUNG reflex area ⑤.

Finally, in the fleshy portion beneath the little toe, is the SHOULDER reflex area ⑥.

These reflex areas appear in the same place on both the left and right foot, with the left foot representing the left side of the body and the right foot representing the right side. Even though the heart is situated on the left-hand side of the body, it has a reflex area on the right foot as well as on the left.

4 Change hands and hold the toes back with the right hand. Begin with the DIAPHRAGM reflex area, using the thumb of the left hand to walk through this segment of the LUNG, CHEST and UPPER BACK reflex areas. Work through the padded ball of the foot and up between the third and fourth toes.

5 Beginning in the DIAPHRAGM reflex area, thumb-walk with your left hand up through the SHOULDER reflex area.

DESSERTS   Side-to-side (p. 68) • Lung press (p. 70) • Sole-mover (p. 71)

STEP 4

Working the upper arch of the foot

The reflex areas in this sequence correspond to organs responsible for producing many of the chemicals needed for digestion, energy and water balance. In addition, the kidneys purify blood and fluid, and other organs produce enzymes to help digest food. To orient yourself, visualise the waistline as being across the middle of the foot and the diaphragm as across the lower edge of the ball of the foot. Work between these areas (*see right*) to stimulate and enhance the function of the organs addressed in this sequence.

AREAS WORKED
PANCREAS: This is responsible for stabilising blood glucose levels.
ADRENAL GLANDS: Working these glands may help regulate levels of hormones, such as adrenaline.
KIDNEYS: Strain fluids in the blood for excretion or absorption.
STOMACH: Aim to assist digestion by targeting this reflex area.
LIVER, GALL BLADDER & SPLEEN: Reflexology may help these organs regulate chemical levels in the blood, excreting the unwanted substances as bile.

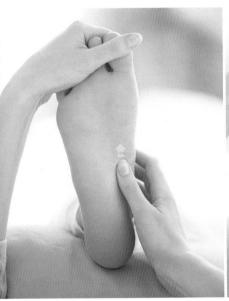

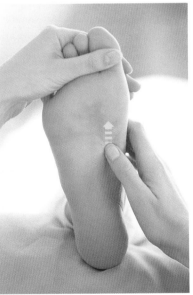

1 Hold the toes back with your left hand and use your right thumb to walk through the PANCREAS reflex area. (On the left foot, the PANCREAS reflex area extends across the foot.)

2 Continue walking with the right thumb up the foot. At the midpoint on the long bone (*see page 41*), you will find the ADRENAL GLAND reflex area and a portion of the STOMACH reflex area. Make several passes.

CAUTION

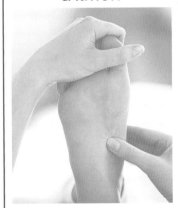

When holding the foot back, take care to avoid applying pressure to the long tendon that runs through this part of the foot. To locate it, hold the toes back and run your thumb lightly down the foot below the ball of the foot. To avoid problems, lessen the stretch of the foot when thumb-walking across the tendon.

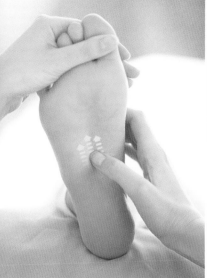

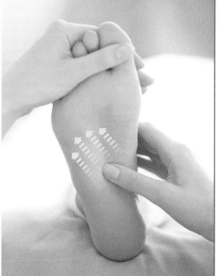

FOOT ORIENTATION

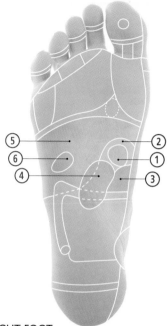

3 Reposition your right thumb on the KIDNEY reflex area. Use the thumb-walking technique to make several passes through this reflex area.

4 Next, beginning at the KIDNEY reflex area, make a series of diagonal passes through the LIVER and GALL BLADDER reflex areas.

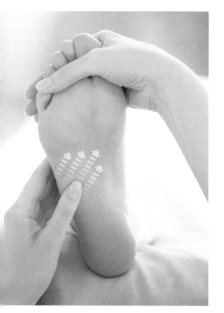

5 Change hands. From the waistline marker, walk your left thumb in the other direction, making another series of diagonal passes through the LIVER and GALL BLADDER reflex areas.

RIGHT FOOT

The reflex areas for organs and glands involved in excretion, absorption and digestion lie on the upper arch of the foot. Many overlap each other (indicated by broken white lines).

The ADRENAL GLANDS reflex area ① is surrounded by the STOMACH area ②. Just underneath lies the reflex area relating to the PANCREAS ③. Next to it is the distinctively shaped KIDNEY reflex area ④. The large LIVER reflex area ⑤ encloses the GALL BLADDER reflex area ⑥.

It is important to note that reflex areas for many of these organs are not the same size or in the same positions on both the left and right foot. For example, the stomach reflex area is much larger on the left foot. In addition, the gall bladder reflex area is only to be found on the right foot and the spleen reflex area only on the left. (*For the location of reflex areas on the left foot, see page 17.*)

DESSERTS   Side-to-side (*p. 68*) • Sole-mover (*p. 71*) • Lung press (*p. 70*)

STEP 5

Working the lower arch of the foot

This sequence addresses reflex areas corresponding to body organs that process food and eliminate waste after digestion. Work the reflex areas listed in this step to encourage the smooth running of the small intestine, the ileocaecal valve and the colon.

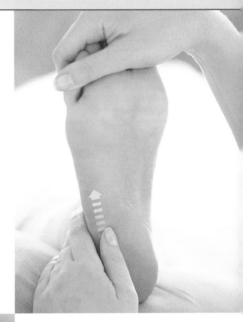

2 Proceed from the ILEOCAECAL VALVE reflex area to the COLON reflex area. Hold the toes back with the right hand, and use the thumb of the left hand to walk up the reflex area for the ASCENDING COLON to that of the TRANSVERSE COLON.

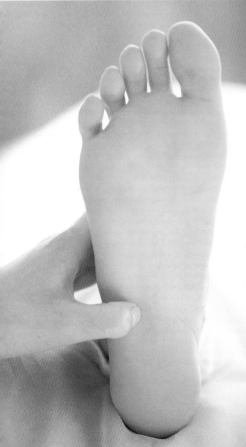

1 To find the ILEOCAECAL VALVE reflex area, run your left hand down the outside of the foot from the fifth metatarsal bone to the heel (*see page 41*). Do you feel the hollow spot along here? The reflex point is located in the deepest part of this hollow (*see left*). Using the hook and back-up technique, hook into this spot and back across it with your thumb.

AREAS WORKED

ILEOCAECAL VALVE: This releases undigested material from the small intestine into the colon.

COLON: Apply reflexology to this area to aid in the storage and expulsion of waste products in the form of faecal matter.

SMALL INTESTINE: Working this reflex area may assist the small intestine in breaking down food.

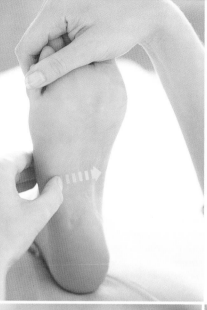

3 Reposition your hand, placing your left thumb at the foot's waistline. Thumb-walk through the TRANSVERSE COLON reflex area, across the centre of the foot.

FOOT ORIENTATION

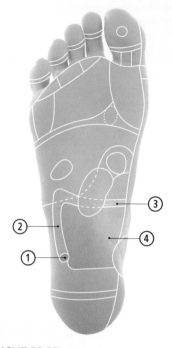

RIGHT FOOT

The reflex areas corresponding to the lower part of the abdomen can be found just above the pad of the heel.

The ILEOCAECAL VALVE reflex area occupies a very small area just above the heel (1). The COLON reflex area runs upward (ascending colon (2)) and then across (transverse colon (3)). The reflex area corresponding to the small intestine (4) is bordered by the colon reflex area.

On the left foot, there is is no reflex area relating to the ileocaecal valve. The colon reflex area on the left foot is a different shape: it runs across, down (descending colon) and dips across the outside of the left foot (sigmoid colon). (*For the location of reflex areas on the left foot, see page 17.*)

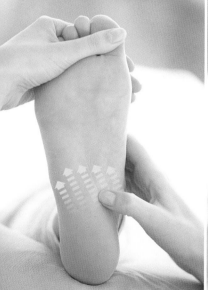

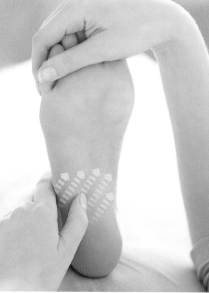

4 Change hands and hold the toes back with the left hand. Walk diagonally upwards with the right thumb across the SMALL INTESTINE reflex area, letting up on the tendon as you pass over it.

5 To work the COLON, change hands and with your left thumb work diagonally across the SMALL INTESTINE reflex area from the other direction, ending your passes in the TRANSVERSE COLON reflex area.

DESSERTS   Toe rotation (*p. 72*) • Traction (*p. 73*) • Mid-foot mover (*p. 73*)

STEP 6

Working the inside of the foot

This sequence works reflex areas such as that of the spine, which runs up the entire inside length of the foot. The steps in this sequence also work the bladder and the point that in women corresponds to the uterus and in men to the prostate gland.

AREAS WORKED

UTERUS/PROSTATE GLAND: The application of reflexology techniques aims to enhance function of the uterus in females and of the prostate gland in males.

SPINE: This reflex area runs the entire length of the inside of the foot, mirroring the way the spine runs downs the torso.

BLADDER: This organ stores urine for excretion.

NECK & BRAIN STEM: Applying reflexology work to this area aims to provide a relaxing effect.

1 Pinpoint the UTERUS/PROSTATE GLAND reflex area. To do this, place the tip of your right index finger on the inside of the ankle bone and the tip of your ring finger on the back corner of the heel. Now draw your middle finger in until it forms a straight line with the others and establishes a midpoint. This is the UTERUS/ PROSTATE GLAND reflex area.

2 Rest your left middle finger on this reflex point, cupping the heel in the palm of your hand. Grasp the ball of the foot with the right hand and apply the rotating on a point technique, turning the foot clockwise in a 360° circle several times.

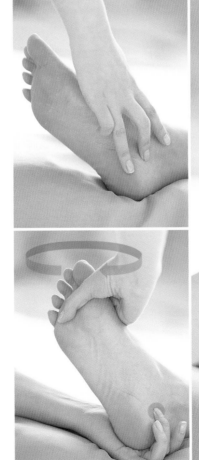

3 Now turn the foot anti-clockwise several times.

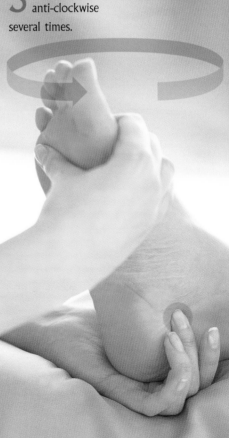

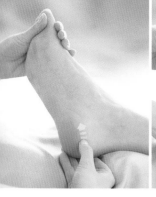 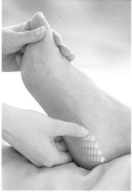 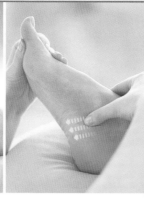

4 Steady the foot with your left hand and use the right thumb to walk through the TAILBONE reflex area. Repeat.

5 To further work the TAILBONE reflex area, reposition your right thumb at the side of the heel and make several passes.

6 Reposition your working thumb at the BLADDER and LOWER BACK reflex areas. Thumb walk through the area several times.

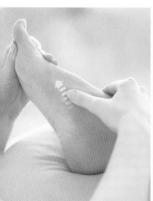 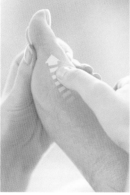 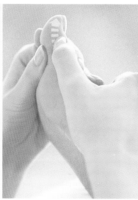

7 Now reposition your working thumb again. Use the thumb-walking technique to walk up the reflex area for the UPPER BACK. Make several passes.

8 Begin thumb-walking at the DIAPHRAGM reflex area, making several passes up through the area representing the part of the SPINE between the shoulder blades.

9 To work the NECK and BRAIN STEM reflex areas, walk up the side of the big toe with your thumb. Once again, you should make several passes.

DESSERTS Side-to-side (p. 68) • Spinal twist (p. 69) • Mid-foot mover (p. 73)

FOOT ORIENTATION

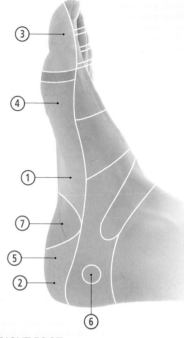

RIGHT FOOT

On the inside of the foot can be found reflex areas corresponding to the spine, reproductive organs and the bladder.

Running the entire length of the inside of the foot is the reflex area for the SPINE (1), with the TAILBONE represented at the heel (2) and the NECK and BRAIN STEM at the the tip of the big toe (3). The UPPER BACK section of the spine reflex area (4) lies above "the waistline marker," which runs horizontally across the middle of the foot, and the LOWER BACK section below the waistline marker (5). The reflex area representing the female UTERUS and male PROSTATE GLAND occupy the same spot just below the ankle (6). Finally, the BLADDER reflex area lies just below the inside of the ankle (7).

The reflex areas on the left and right feet mirror each other, with areas on the left foot corresponding to the left side of the body, and those on the right foot relating to the right.

STEP 7

Working the tops of the toes

This sequence works those areas of the body responsible for musculo-skeletal activities like chewing and turning the head. These include reflex areas for the face, sinuses, neck, teeth, jaw and gums. To orient yourself, visualise your head and neck spanning the tops of the toes. Work these reflex points to stimulate and enhance function in corresponding body parts and to relax tension.

AREAS WORKED
FACE & SINUS: Control and co-ordinate all activity in the body, so a key part of a reflexology session.
NECK: Highly prone to tension, it may respond well to reflexology.
TEETH, JAWS & GUMS: The effectiveness of this network of tissue and bone responsible for breaking down food in the mouth may be promoted by reflexology.

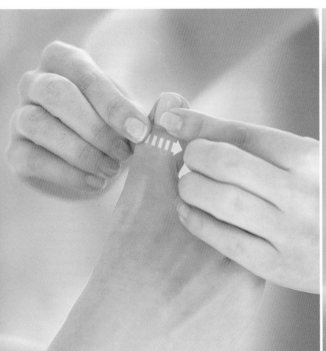

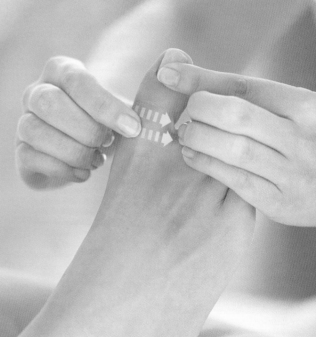

1 Start by anchoring the big toe with the fingertips and thumb of your left hand. Beginning below the toenail, walk your right index finger round the FACE and SINUS reflex areas. Make a series of passes across the top of the toe under the nail.

2 Repositioning your index finger, walk the right index finger forward in a series of passes round the base of the big toe, the NECK reflex area.

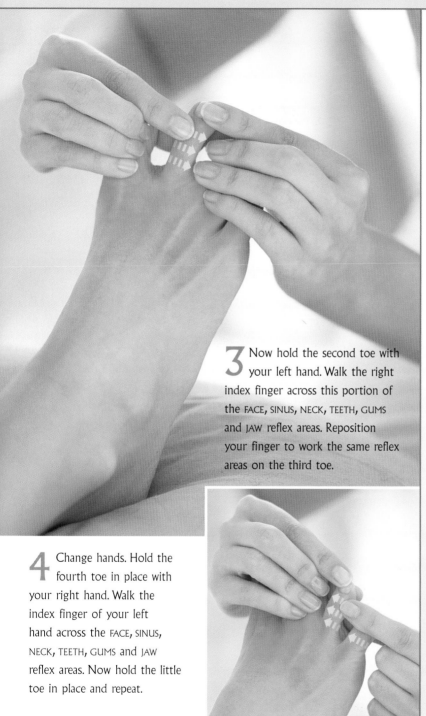

FOOT ORIENTATION

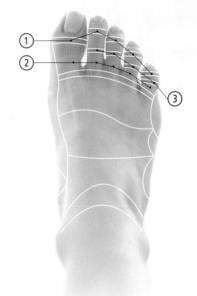

3 Now hold the second toe with your left hand. Walk the right index finger across this portion of the FACE, SINUS, NECK, TEETH, GUMS and JAW reflex areas. Reposition your finger to work the same reflex areas on the third toe.

4 Change hands. Hold the fourth toe in place with your right hand. Walk the index finger of your left hand across the FACE, SINUS, NECK, TEETH, GUMS and JAW reflex areas. Now hold the little toe in place and repeat.

RIGHT FOOT

The tops of the toes can be seen as mirroring the face, with the sinuses, teeth, jaw and gums all represented, and with the reflex area for the neck lying in the joint of each toe where it attaches to the foot.

The reflex area for the FACE and SINUS is a band that runs across the first joint of each of the toes ①. The fleshy segments of each of the toes, below the first joint, represent the NECK ②. The middle joint of each toe corresponds to the TEETH, GUMS and JAW ③.

The reflex areas on the left foot exactly mirror those on the right, with the reflex areas on the right foot representing the right side of the body, and those on the left corresponding to the left side of the body.

DESSERTS Traction (p. 73) • Toe rotation (p. 72) • Mid-foot mover (p. 73)

STEP 8

Working the top of the foot

The reflex areas in this step correspond to areas of the body responsible for respiration, milk production and reproduction. The main areas worked also overlap with those of the upper torso, so working these particular reflex points relaxes musculo-skeletal tension in the upper body as well as stimulating and enhancing function in the primary areas treated.

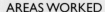

AREAS WORKED
CHEST & LUNGS: Reflexology work here may help loosen catarrh.
BREAST: Working this reflex may help regulate breast milk production.
UPPER BACK: Working this reflex area may ease tension in the upper torso.
LOWER BACK: Working this reflex area may ease pain in this part of the back.
LYMPH GLANDS: Aim to drain lymph from the body and bolster immunity by working this area.
GROIN & FALLOPIAN TUBES: These areas may respond well to reflexology.

1 Holding the foot upright with your left hand, open up the "trough" along the top of the foot by spreading the toes apart. Starting at the base of the big toe, walk your right index finger through the first segment of the LUNG, CHEST, BREAST and UPPER BACK reflex areas. You will feel a long bone as you finger-walk down to the waistline marker.

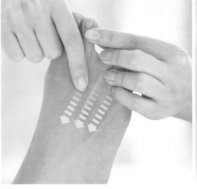

2 To work the second segment of the LUNG, CHEST, BREAST and UPPER BACK reflex areas, spread the second and third toes apart and finger-walk through this area. Repeat on the areas between the third and fourth toes, finger-walking down each segment of this reflex area, then repeat the sequence between the fourth and fifth toes.

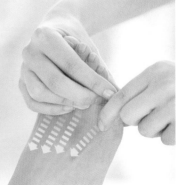

3 Now change hands to work through the other side of each trough. Spread the fourth and fifth toes apart with your right hand. Apply the finger-walking technique with your left hand. Work the rest of the troughs in the same manner.

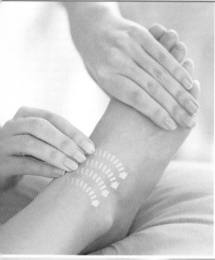

4 Hold the foot steady with your left hand. Rest your fingers on top of the foot in the SPINE reflex area. Using all four fingers together, finger-walk through the LOWER BACK reflex area.

FOOT ORIENTATION

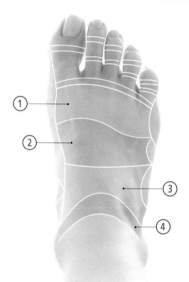

5 Now, hold the foot upright with your right hand. Using your left hand, thumb-walk through the reflex areas for the FALLOPIAN TUBES, LYMPH GLANDS and GROIN.

This step may also be done using both thumbs simultaneously.

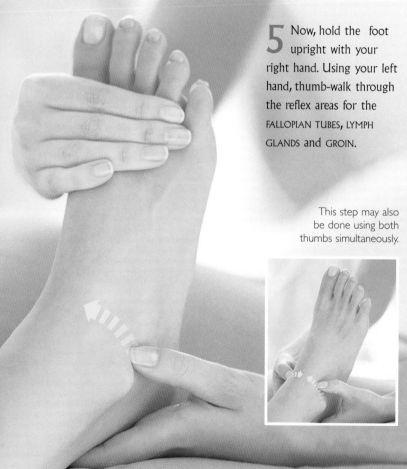

RIGHT FOOT

The top of the foot contains a number of important reflex areas which run in horizontal bands across it.

The LUNG, CHEST, BREAST and UPPER BACK reflex area form a broad band on the tops of the feet, below the toes ①. Moving up the foot, the area corresponding to the rest of the UPPER BACK also runs across the foot in a horizontal block ②. The reflex area for the LOWER BACK is in a third band ③. Finally, the reflex areas for the FALLOPIAN TUBES, LYMPH GLANDS and GROIN are found in a crescent band around the ankle where it meets the top of the foot ④.

The reflex areas on the left and right feet mirror each other perfectly, with those on the right foot corresponding to the right half of the body and those on the left relating to the left half of the body.

DESSERTS   Lung press (p. 70) • Sole-mover (p. 71) • Ankle rotation (p. 72)

STEP 9

Working the outside of the foot

The reflex areas in this step correspond to many of the body's joints, limbs and reproductive organs. This includes the hip, sciatic nerve, knee, leg, arm, elbow and the ovaries in women or the testicles in men. Work these reflex areas to improve functioning of these parts of the body. Follow this sequence by applying a series of desserts to relax the foot, and end it with a final resting position. After working through the left foot, end your workout with a relaxing finish, the breathing technique.

AREAS WORKED
SCIATIC NERVES: These nerves run down the back of each thigh.
HIPS, LEGS & KNEES: Apply techniques to these reflex areas to facilitate mobility.
ARMS & ELBOWS: Prone to stiffness, the limb of the upper body and its central joint may respond well to reflexology.
OVARIES & TESTICLES: To enhance function of the female and male sex organs, use reflexology techniques regularly.

1 Start by holding the foot upright with your left hand. Use the index finger of the right hand to walk round the ankle bone and through the HIP and SCIATIC NERVE reflex areas.

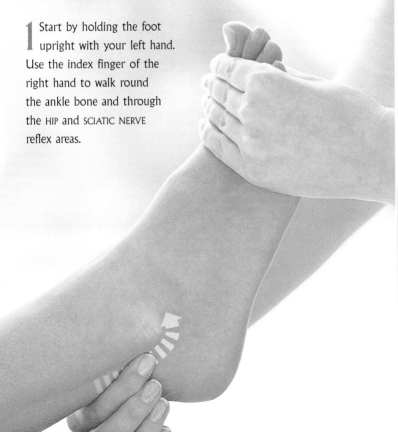

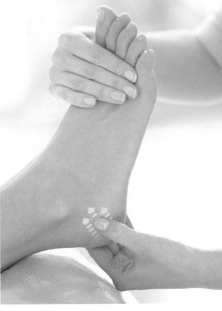

2 Change hands, holding the foot steady with the right hand. Use the left thumb to walk through the OVARY / TESTICLE area.

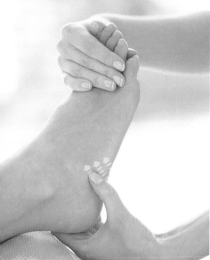

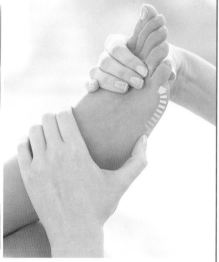

3 Next, thumb-walk through the KNEE and LEG reflex areas, making a series of passes.

4 Now reposition your left hand. Starting from the KNEE and LEG reflex areas, thumb-walk up the ELBOW and ARM reflex areas.

DESSERTS   Side-to-side (p. 68) • Spinal twist (p. 69) • Lung press (p. 70) • Ankle rotation (p. 72)

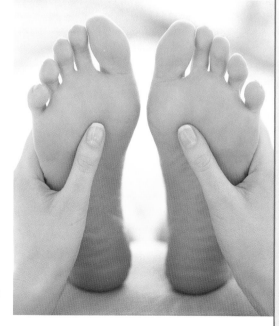

Breathing: Place your thumbs in the SOLAR PLEXUS reflex areas of each foot. Press slightly while the recipient takes three deep breaths.

FOOT ORIENTATION

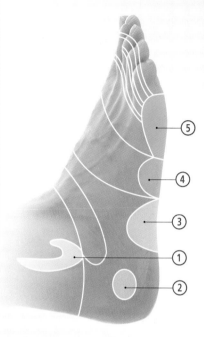

RIGHT FOOT

On the outside edge of the foot can be found reflex areas relating to both the limbs and to the male and female reproductive organs.

On the underside of the ankle bone, lies the reflex area for the HIP and the SCIATIC NERVE ①. Nearby, the reflex area for the OVARY in women and the TESTICLE in men can be found on the outside edge of the heel ②. On the edge of the foot, in a semi-circle, is the area corresponding to the KNEE and LEG ③. Moving up the foot, is the reflex area for the ELBOW ④ and finally on the fleshy pad of the little toe is the reflex area for the ARM ⑤.

These reflex areas all appear in the same place on both the left and the right foot, with the left foot representing the left arm and elbow, for example, and the right foot relating to the right-hand side of the body.

STEP 10
Working the left foot

Now that you've given the right foot a workout, it's time to move on to the left foot. These pages show the sequence for a left-foot workout. They also provide a workout summary. Once you have become familiar with how techniques are applied to each part of the foot, this summary provides an at-a-glance reminder of reflexology technique applications.

DESSERTS

Before beginning the sequence, check the foot fo cuts, bruises and areas to b avoided when working

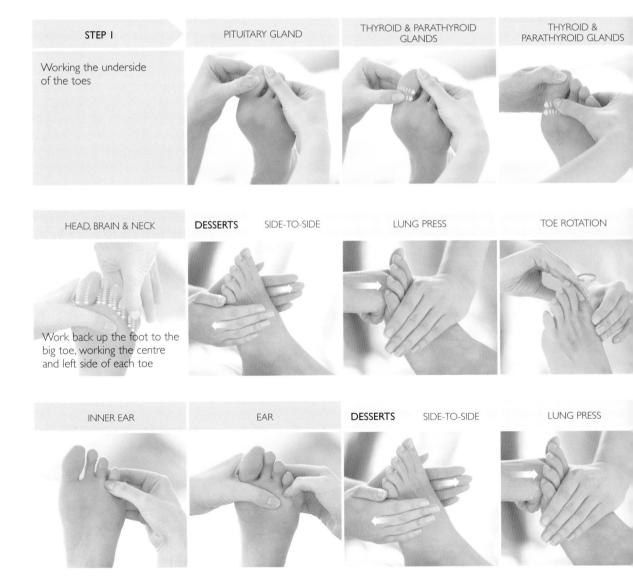

STEP I	PITUITARY GLAND	THYROID & PARATHYROID GLANDS	THYROID & PARATHYROID GLANDS

Working the underside of the toes

HEAD, BRAIN & NECK	DESSERTS SIDE-TO-SIDE	LUNG PRESS	TOE ROTATION

Work back up the foot to the big toe, working the centre and left side of each toe

INNER EAR	EAR	DESSERTS SIDE-TO-SIDE	LUNG PRESS

SIDE-TO-SIDE

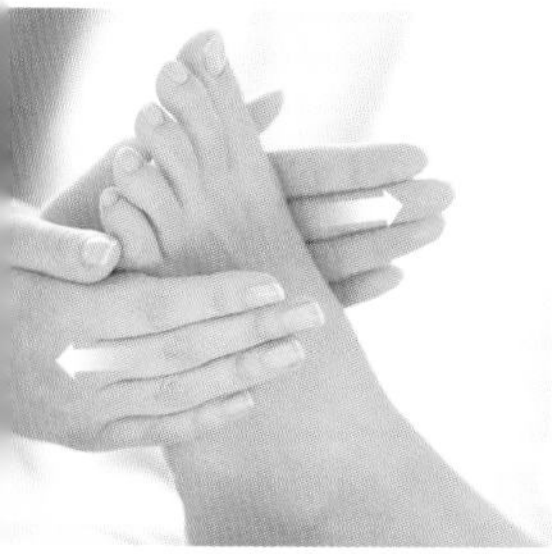

SPINAL TWIST

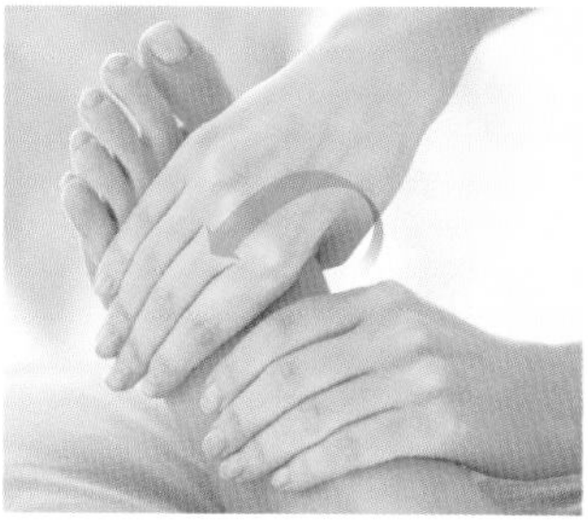

LUNG PRESS

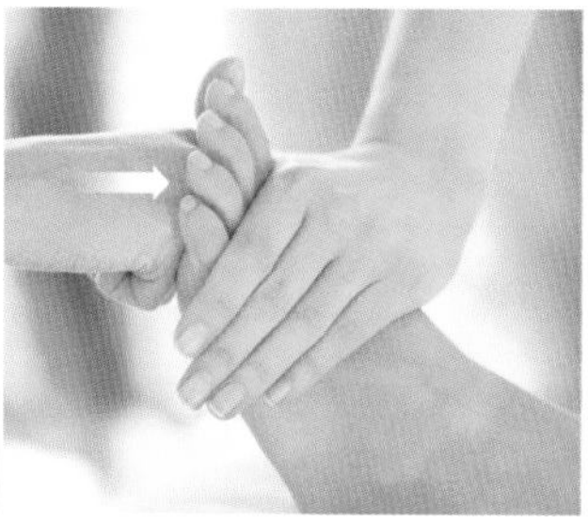

TOE ROTATION

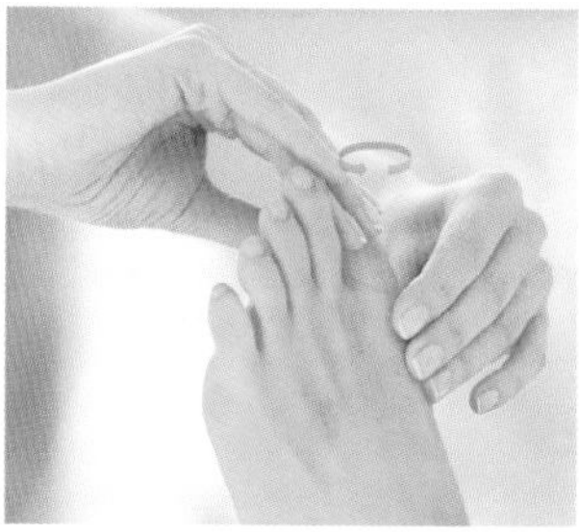

HEAD, BRAIN & NECK

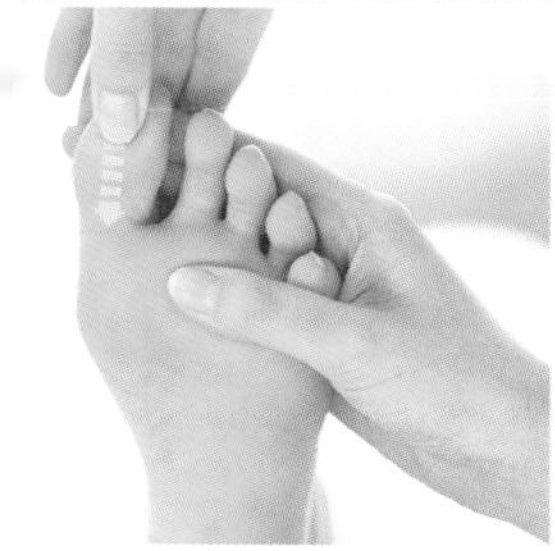

HEAD, BRAIN & NECK

HEAD, BRAIN & NECK

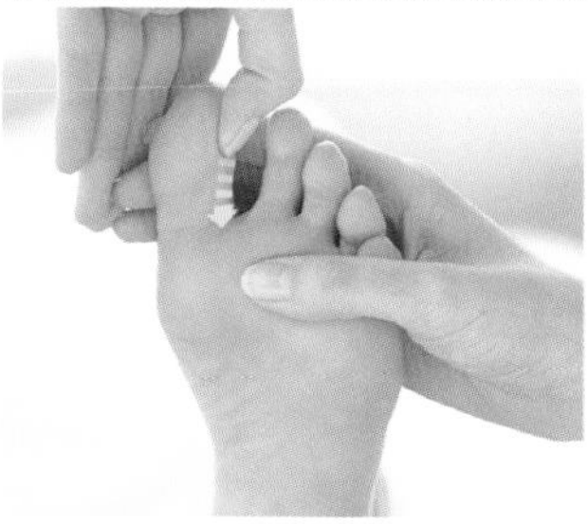

HEAD, BRAIN & NECK

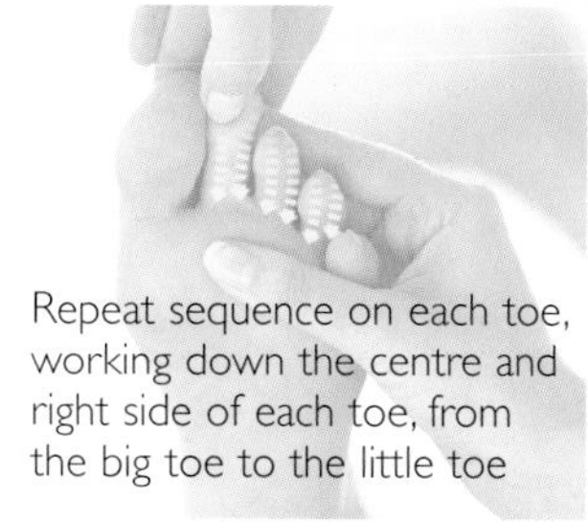

Repeat sequence on each toe, working down the centre and right side of each toe, from the big toe to the little toe

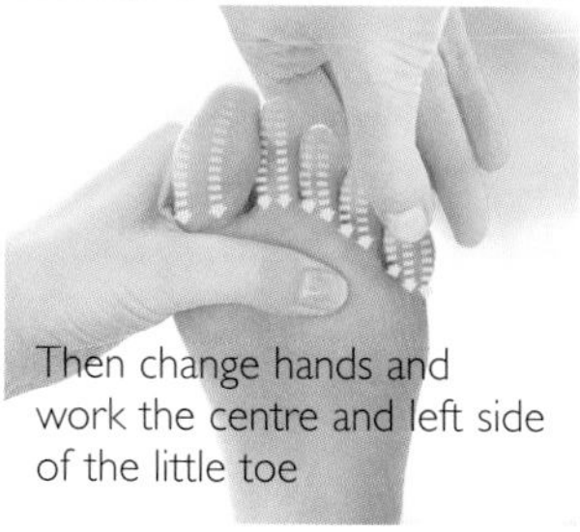

Then change hands and work the centre and left side of the little toe

STEP 2

Working the base of the toes

EYE, EAR & INNER EAR

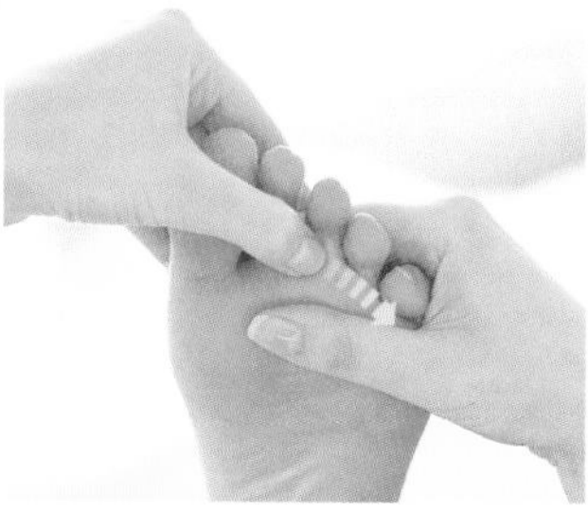

EYE, EAR & INNER EAR

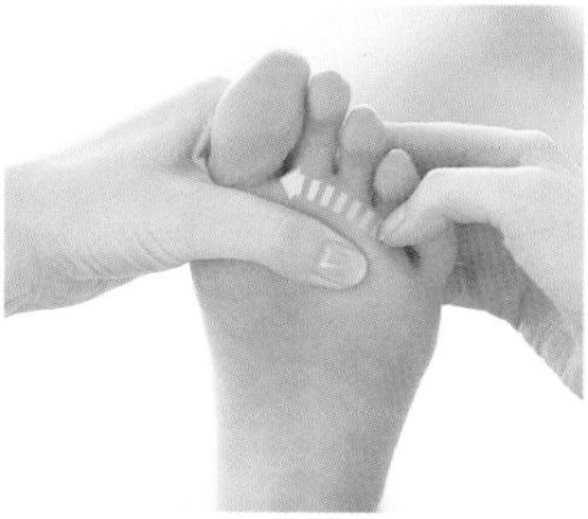

EYE

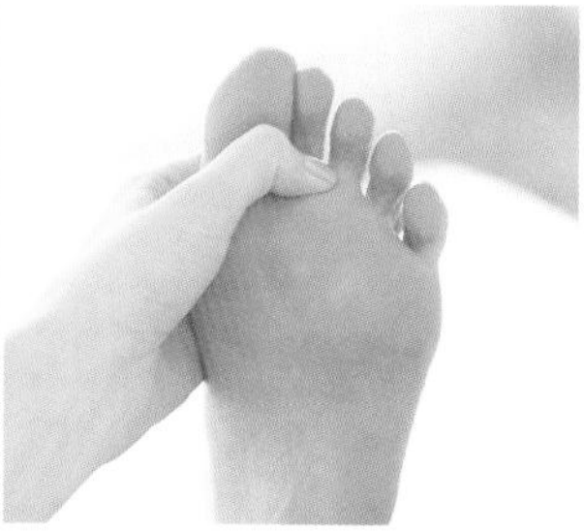

SOLE-MOVER

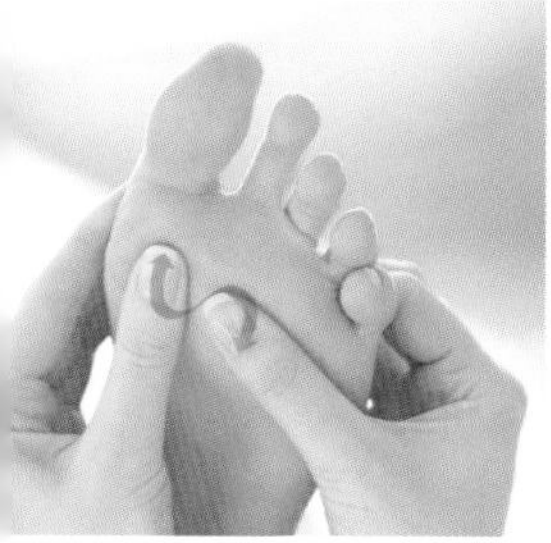

STEP 3

Working the ball of the foot

HEART & CHEST

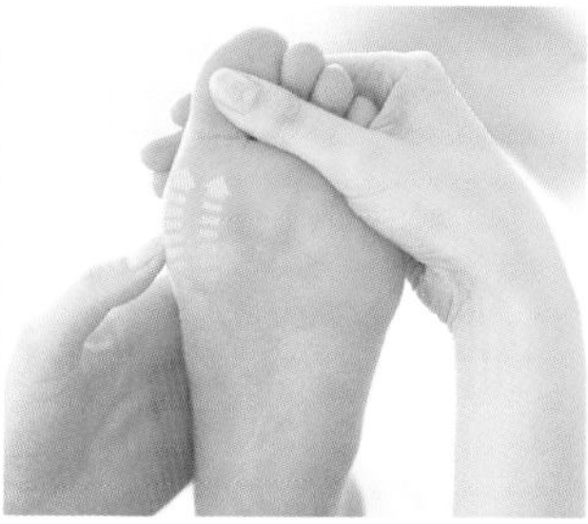

SOLAR PLEXUS

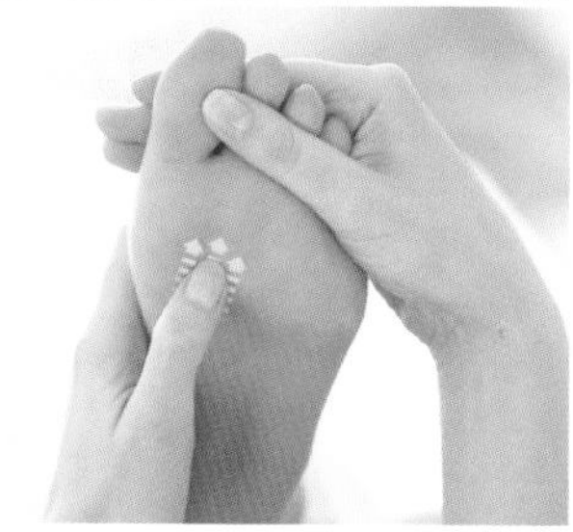

LUNG, CHEST & UPPER BACK	LUNG, CHEST & UPPER BACK	SHOULDER	**DESSERTS** SIDE-TO-SIDE

ADRENAL GLAND & STOMACH	KIDNEY	LIVER & SPLEEN	LIVER & SPLEEN

TRANSVERSE COLON	DESCENDING COLON	SIGMOID COLON	SMALL INTESTINE

STEP 6	UTERUS/PROSTATE GLAND	UTERUS/PROSTATE GLAND	UTERUS/PROSTATE GLAND

STEP 6

Working the inside of the foot

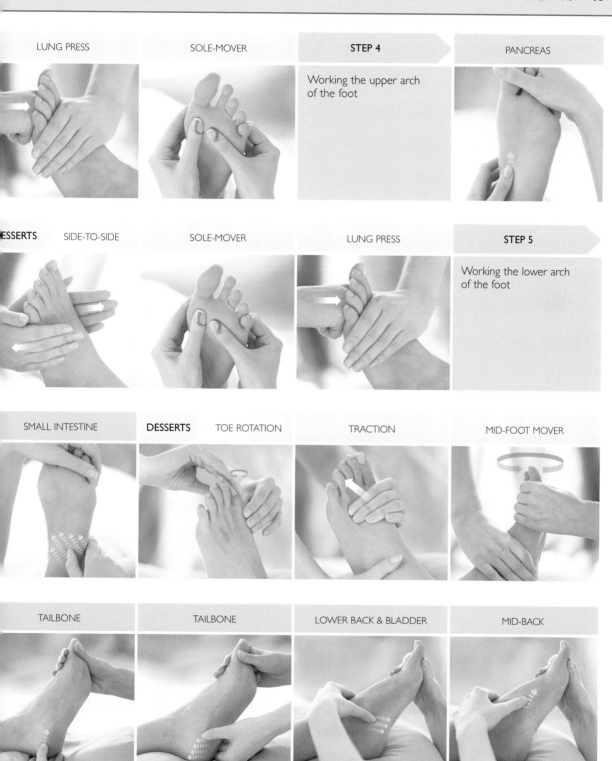

LUNG PRESS

SOLE-MOVER

STEP 4

Working the upper arch
of the foot

PANCREAS

ESSERTS   SIDE-TO-SIDE

SOLE-MOVER

LUNG PRESS

STEP 5

Working the lower arch
of the foot

SMALL INTESTINE

DESSERTS   TOE ROTATION

TRACTION

MID-FOOT MOVER

TAILBONE

TAILBONE

LOWER BACK & BLADDER

MID-BACK

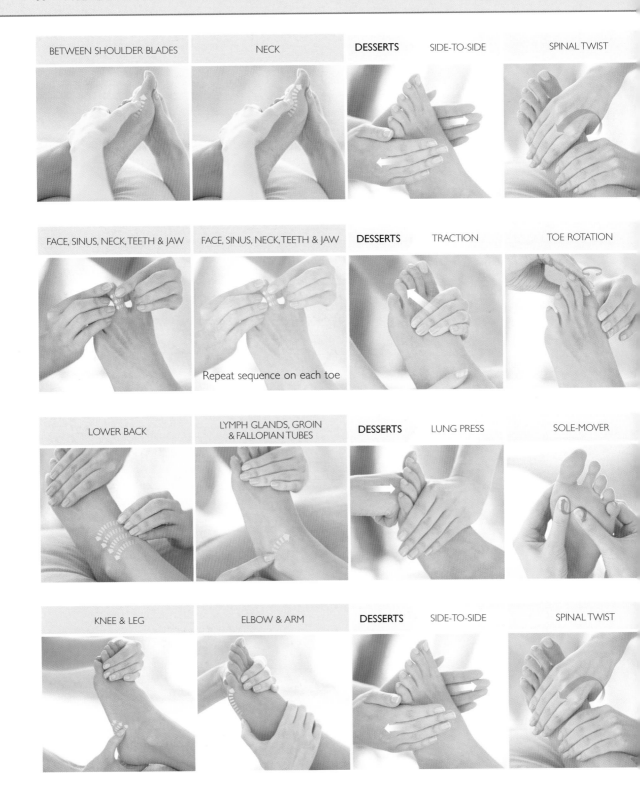

| BETWEEN SHOULDER BLADES | NECK | DESSERTS   SIDE-TO-SIDE | SPINAL TWIST |

| FACE, SINUS, NECK, TEETH & JAW | FACE, SINUS, NECK, TEETH & JAW | DESSERTS   TRACTION | TOE ROTATION |

Repeat sequence on each toe

| LOWER BACK | LYMPH GLANDS, GROIN & FALLOPIAN TUBES | DESSERTS   LUNG PRESS | SOLE-MOVER |

| KNEE & LEG | ELBOW & ARM | DESSERTS   SIDE-TO-SIDE | SPINAL TWIST |

MID-FOOT MOVER	STEP 7	HEAD & BRAIN	NECK

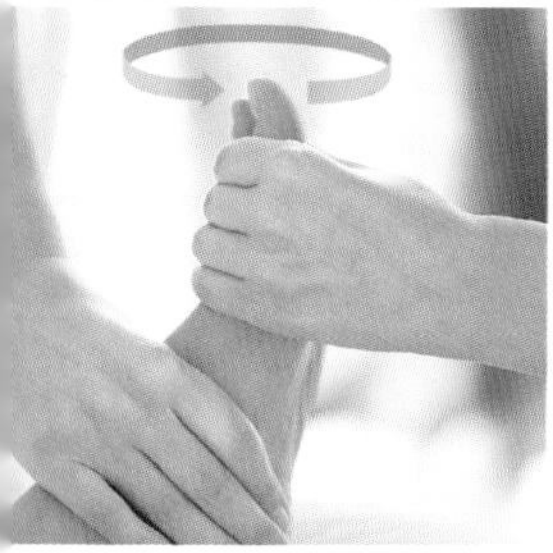

Working the tops of the toes

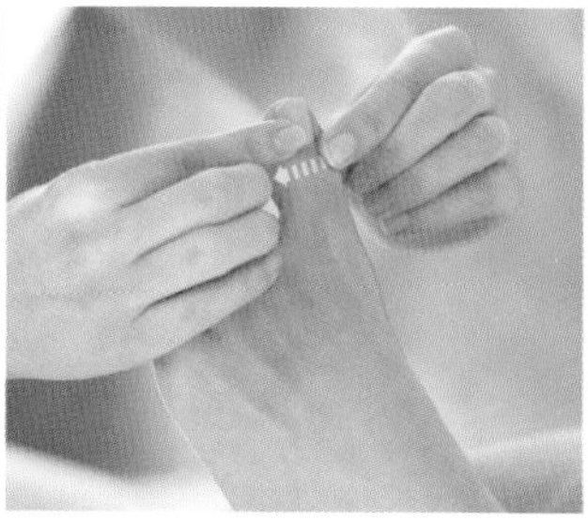

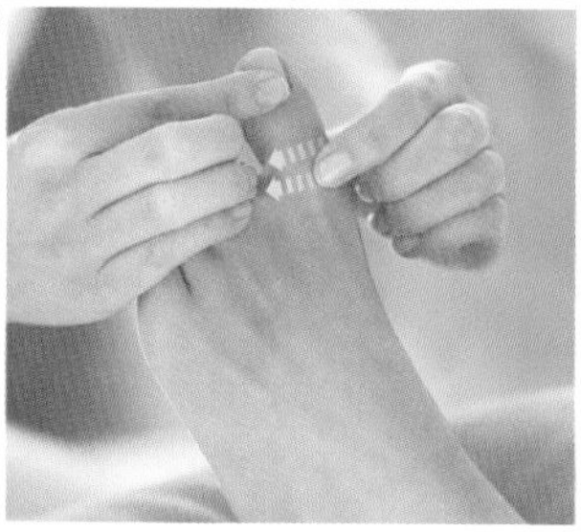

MID-FOOT MOVER	STEP 8	LUNG, CHEST & BREAST	LUNG, CHEST & BREAST

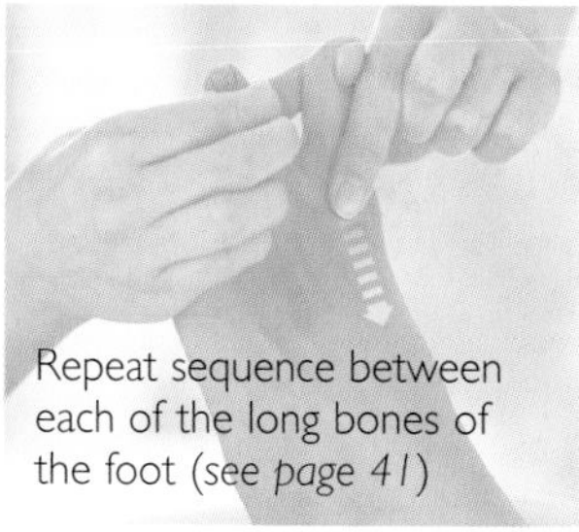

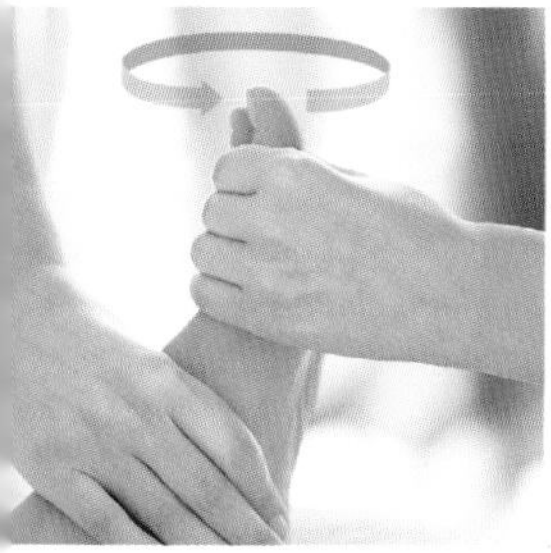

Working the top of the foot

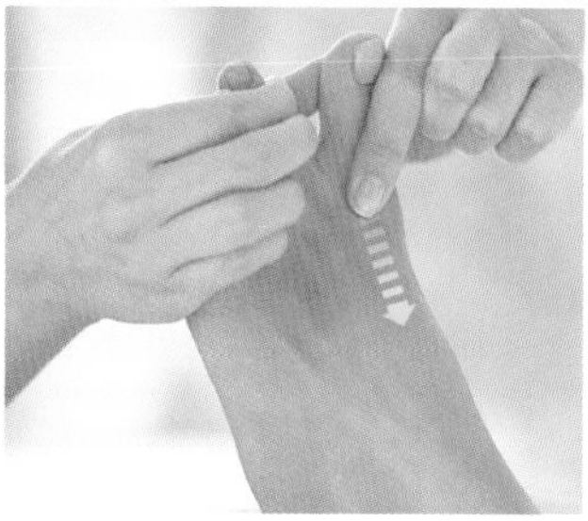

Repeat sequence between each of the long bones of the foot (see page 41)

ANKLE ROTATION	STEP 9	HIP & SCIATIC NERVE	OVARY/TESTICLE

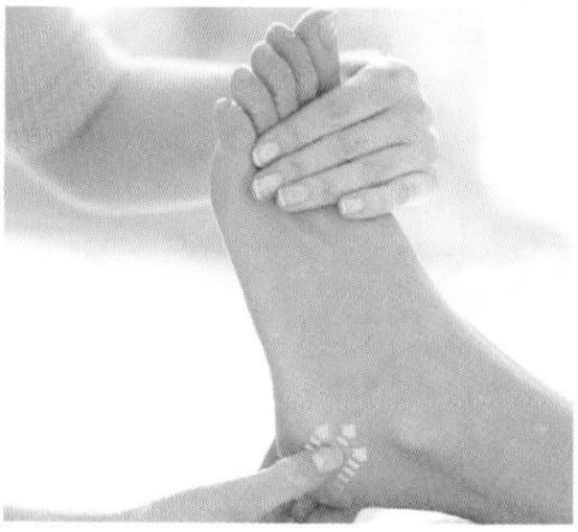

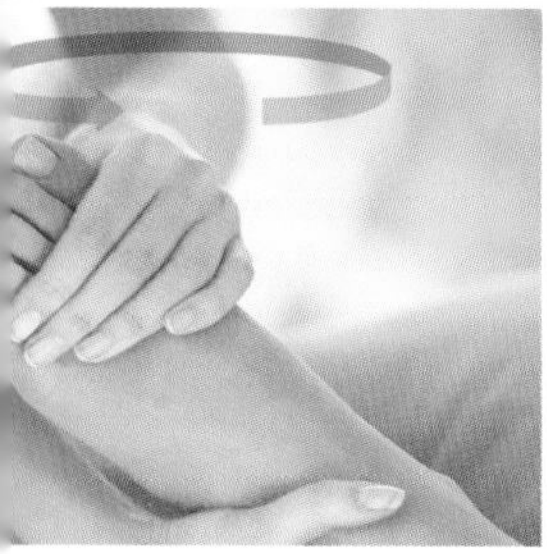

Working the outside of the foot

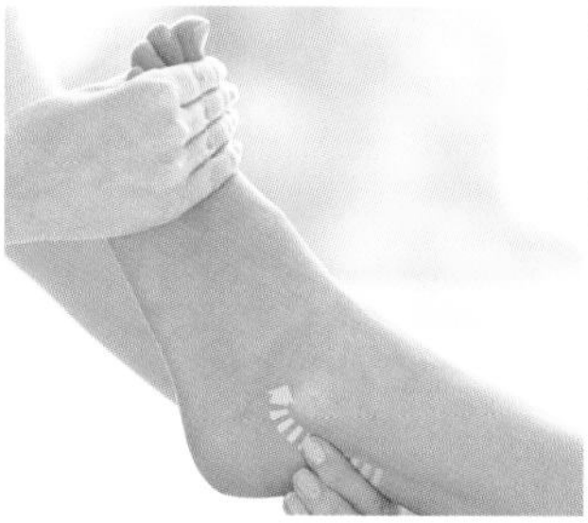

LUNG PRESS	ANKLE ROTATION	BREATHING

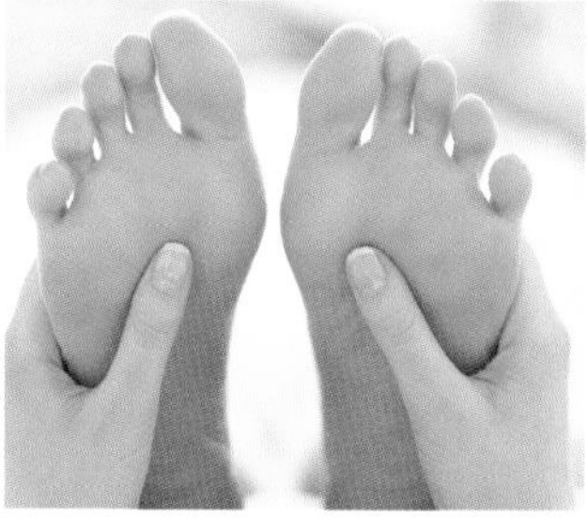

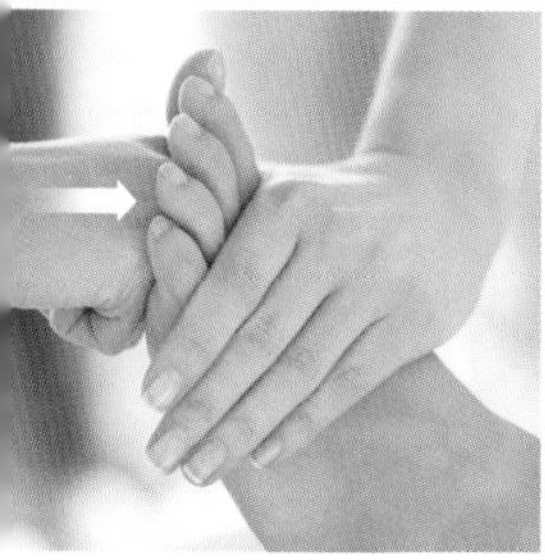

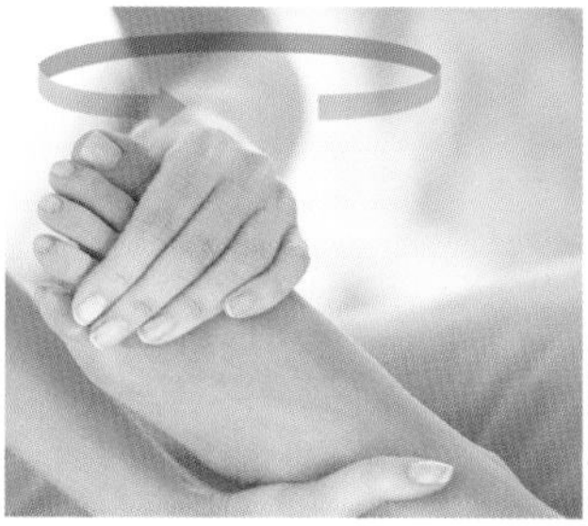

HAND DESSERTS

There are several hand reflexology dessert techniques
that relax the hand and explore its flexibility and range
of movement. Techniques such as the finger-pull, the walk-
down / pull-against, the palm-rocker and the hand-stretcher
provide a beginning, an end and a transition between
techniques. Some hand desserts may feature thumb-walking,
so simply apply to the hand the basic thumb-walking
technique described earlier in this chapter (*see page 62*).

Finger-pull

The finger-pull technique creates "traction",
which is an easy way to relax not just the fingers
but the whole hand. During the day, the fingers are
commonly subject to compression. This gentle pull
loosens the joints and relieves compression.

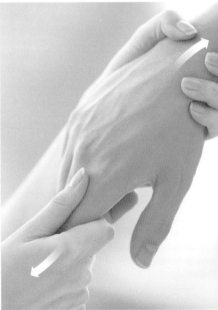

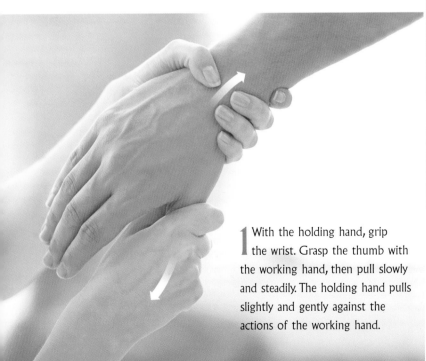

1 With the holding hand, grip
the wrist. Grasp the thumb with
the working hand, then pull slowly
and steadily. The holding hand pulls
slightly and gently against the
actions of the working hand.

2 Change the position of
the holding hand slightly
(*see above*). Apply the pull
technique to the index finger,
then repeat this pattern on
each of the other fingers.

Finger side-to-side

The goal of this technique is to move the finger joints in a way that is different to normal. The working hand creates a slight side-to-side movement, while the holding hand keeps the finger steady.

1 To use this technique, grip the thumb (*see right*). The holding hand grips the joint of the thumb nearest the hand, keeping the upper joint static. With your working hand, move the lower joint of the thumb from side to side. Repeat this movement several times.

2 Move to the index finger and repeat, then repeat with each finger.

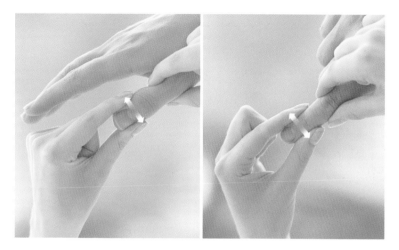

Walk-down / pull-against

This technique stretches the fingers and the thumb. Holding the hand steady, you thumb-walk with the other hand, to create a comfortable, enhanced stretch. Drop the wrist to weigh down the fingers, stretching the inside of the thumb to be worked, and providing leverage for the working hand.

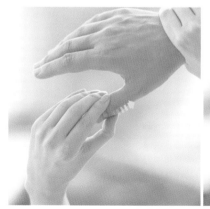
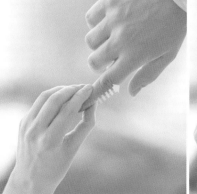
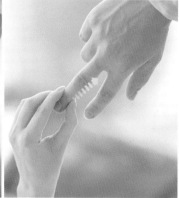

1 Position the working thumb and fingers (*see above*). Make several thumb-walking passes up the outside of the thumb, while stretching the inside of the thumb. Target the joint especially.

2 Move on to the index finger, positioning the working thumb on the side of the finger. Thumb-walk up the outside of the finger, while stretching the inside edge. Repeat several times.

3 Repeat this sequence on each of the fingers in turn several times to stretch the fingers.

Palm-rocker

This dessert creates a rhythmic movement between the long bones of the hand by moving them back and forth alternately. This relaxes the hand, making it more receptive to reflexology work.

1 Grasp the hand (*see right*). Push with the flat of the right thumb and pull with the flat of the index finger of the left hand. Then push with the left thumb and pull with the index finger of the right hand. Repeat several times.

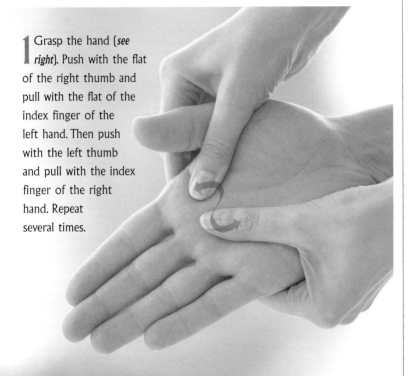

2 Repeat this sequence with the other long bones of the hand (*see page 41*).

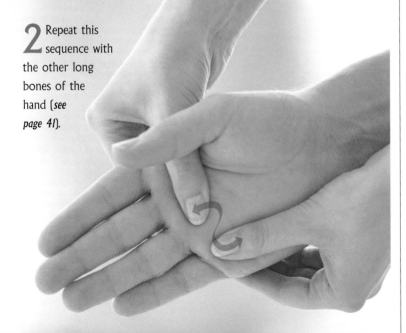

Hand-stretcher

This dessert creates a feeling of relaxation in the body of the hand by stretching the palms.

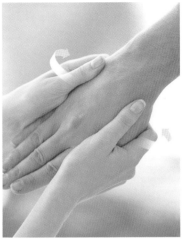

1 Grasp the hand (*see above*). Turn your wrists outwards, pressing up on the palm with your fingers.

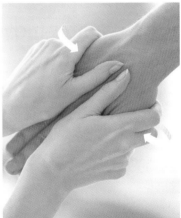

2 Counter this movement by then turning your wrists inwards, pressing against top of the hand with your palms. Repeat these two actions alternately several times.

Palm-mover

This technique is akin to the wringing of the hands. Like the palm rocker (*see opposite*), the goal of the technique is to move the long bones of the hand to promote relaxation.

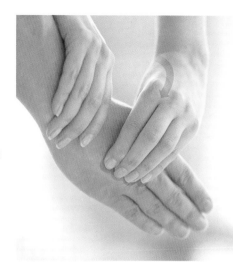

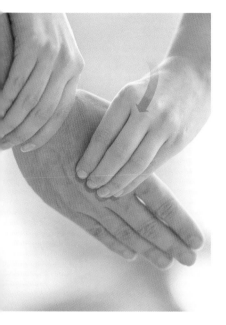

1 Hold the hand steady at the wrist (*see left*). Press gently along the long bone of the index finger on top of the hand with the working fingers. As you do this, create a twisting counter-movement by simultaneously pulling up with the thumb, then release. Repeat the action several times.

2 Move to the long bone of the ring finger. Press with the fingers while simultaneously creating counter-movement by pulling up with the thumb. Release and repeat several times, then repeat the sequence on the long bones of the other fingers.

Palm counter-mover

This technique provides another way of creating movement in the long bones of the hand. It promotes movement from the opposite direction to that of the palm-mover.

1 Grasp the hand at the wrist (*see right*). Rest your working thumb on the top of the hand, on the knuckle of the index finger. Push downwards with your thumb and simultaneously pull with the working hand to twist the outside of the hand upwards. Release and repeat several times.

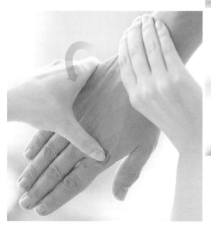

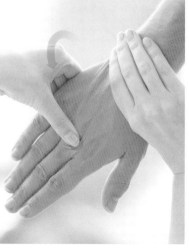

2 Repeat several times on each of the knuckles along the top of the hand in turn.

STEP 1

Working the fingers and the thumb

The areas worked in this sequence, such as the brain, thyroid, parathyroid and pituitary gland, direct many of the body's activites. Work these reflex areas on the hand to stimulate and enhance the functioning of corresponding parts of the body. Before starting the sequence, examine the hand for any areas of injury that should be avoided, and then apply a series of desserts.

DESSERTS   Finger-pull (p. 98) • Finger side-to-side (p. 99) •
Walk-down/pull-against (p. 99) • Hand-stretcher (p. 100)

AREAS WORKED

PITUITARY GLAND: This helps regulate endocrine activity such as growth and metabolism.

NECK: Highly prone to tension, it may respond well to reflexology.

THYROID & PARATHYROID GLANDS: Help to regulate energy levels, metabolism, growth and blood calcium levels. Pressure is applied to these reflex areas to enhance the functions of these glands.

HEAD & BRAIN: Control and co-ordinate all activity in the body, so a key part of a reflexology session.

SINUSES: Reflexology work aims to keep these air-filled cavities clear.

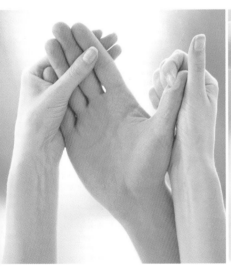

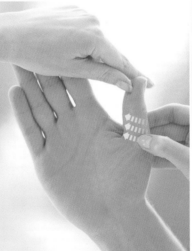

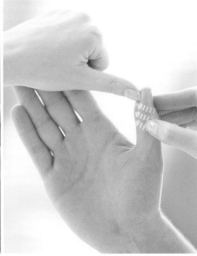

1 To work the PITUITARY GLAND reflex area, hold the hand steady and draw the fingers back with your left hand. Now use your right index finger to repeatedly press the centre of the thumb.

2 Next, hold the thumb with your left hand to steady it. Starting at the base of the thumb, use the thumb-walking technique to make a succession of passes across the thumb through the THYROID / PARATHYROID GLAND and NECK reflex areas.

3 Now make a series of passes higher up at the top of the thumb under the nail to work the HEAD, SINUS and BRAIN reflex areas.

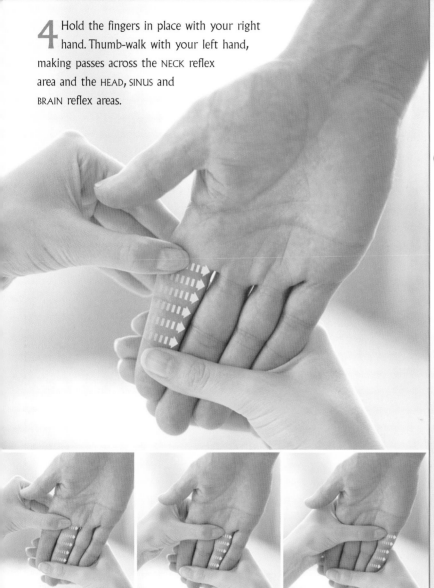

4 Hold the fingers in place with your right hand. Thumb-walk with your left hand, making passes across the NECK reflex area and the HEAD, SINUS and BRAIN reflex areas.

5 Work these reflex areas on the middle finger in the same way.

6 Move on to the ring finger and apply the same series of passes.

7 Finally, apply the same technique series to the reflex areas on the little finger.

DESSERTS Finger-pull (p. 98) • Finger side-to-side (p. 99) • Walk-down/pull-against (p. 99) • Hand-stretcher (p. 100)

HAND ORIENTATION

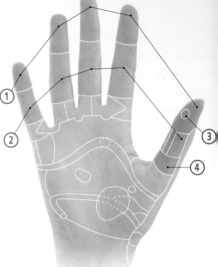

RIGHT HAND

By working reflex areas on the fingers and thumb, this section targets parts of the body round the head and neck.

The tip of each digit has a reflex area corresponding to the HEAD, BRAIN and SINUSES **(1)**. Below this, in the padded flesh under the first joint on each finger and thumb, is a reflex area for the NECK **(2)**. The thumb, as well as having the reflex areas found on the fingers, contains two other reflex areas. In the centre of its fleshy pad you can find the reflex area for the PITUITARY GLAND **(3)**, and at its base is the area representing the THYROID and PARATHYROID GLANDS **(4)**.

The reflex areas on the left hand exactly mirror those on the right, with the left hand relating to the left side of the body, and the right hand corresponding to the right.

STEP 2

Working the thumb and webbing

This sequence is designed to stimulate the parts of the body that produce many of the chemicals needed for digestion, energy and water balance. These areas are also partly responsible for the purification of blood and fluid, as well as the digestion of food. Work these reflex areas on the hand to enhance the functioning of their corresponding body areas. Modify the strength of your action according to the receiver's comfort level.

AREAS WORKED
ADRENAL GLANDS: Working these may help regulate levels of hormones, including adrenaline.
PANCREAS: This is responsible for stabilising blood glucose levels.
STOMACH: Aim to assist digestion by targeting this reflex area.
UPPER BACK: Working this area may ease tension in the upper torso.
KIDNEYS: Strain fluids in the blood for excretion or absorption.

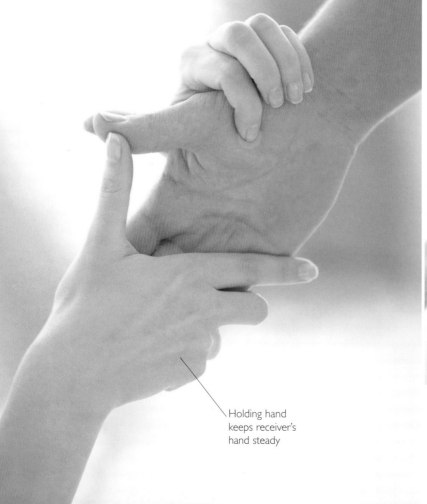

Holding hand keeps receiver's hand steady

1 Start by holding back the fingers and thumb with the right hand. To find the ADRENAL GLAND reflex area, place the tip of your left index finger in the centre of the fleshy palm, midway along the long bone below the thumb. A reaction of sensitivity will indicate that you've found the reflex area. Exert pressure repeatedly with the tip of the finger.

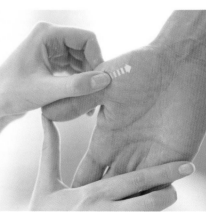

2 Now thumb-walk through the PANCREAS reflex area with your left thumb.

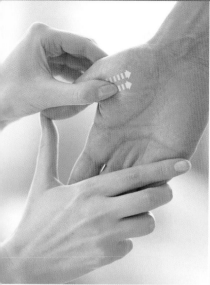

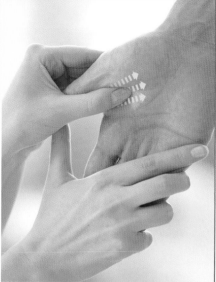

HAND ORIENTATION

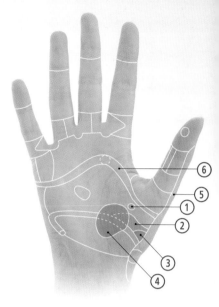

3 Move on, repositioning the left thumb to apply a series of passes throughout the STOMACH reflex area.

4 To work the UPPER BACK and KIDNEY reflex areas, position the left thumb in the webbing of the hand. Apply the thumb-walking technique in successive passes throughout the webbing and into the body of the hand.

RIGHT HAND

Working the reflex areas in the centre and in the fleshy heel of the palm targets a number of internal organs as well as the upper back.

The areas corresponding to the ADRENAL GLANDS ①, STOMACH ②, PANCREAS ③ and KIDNEYS ④ are grouped together – in a similar manner to the way these organs are grouped in the body itself. The UPPER BACK reflex area lies close by on the edge of the palm ⑤, and above the DIAPHRAGM ⑥ reflex area.

5 Next, to work the KIDNEY reflex area more thoroughly, position the left thumb and index finger on opposite sides of the hand. Press into the KIDNEY reflex area on the webbing. Hold for several seconds. Reposition and press again. Find the most sensitive area and apply pressure, modifying the strength of your action according to comfort level.

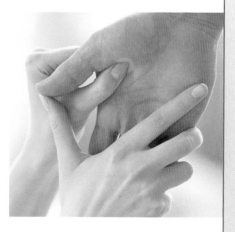

The reflex areas on the left hand exactly mirror those on the right, with the right hand relating to the right side of the body and the left hand corresponding to the left, except where the reflex areas relate to the stomach and pancreas. For both of these, the reflex areas on the right hand are much smaller than those on the left.

DESSERTS   Finger-pull (p. 98) • Hand-stretcher (p. 100) • Palm-mover (p. 101)

STEP 3

Working the upper palm

In this sequence you work areas that correspond to parts of the upper body, including those responsible for providing the body with oxygen and blood, along with those relating to the musculo-skeletal structure of the chest and upper back. Reflex areas for the eye, inner ear and ear are also worked in this step, as they lie directly over the shoulder reflex areas.

AREAS WORKED

HEART: Targeting this reflex area is thought to help to keep the heart functioning well.

CHEST & LUNGS: Apply reflexology to these reflex areas to help keep the chest and lungs open.

UPPER BACK & SHOULDERS: Working these reflex areas may ease tension in the upper torso and the shoulders.

EYES: Reflexology may help soothe sore eyes.

EARS: The application of reflexology techniques may help ease an ear-ache or tinnitus.

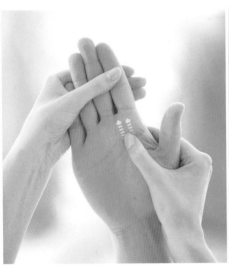

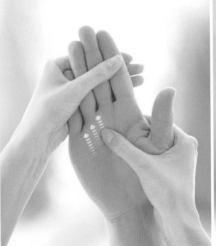

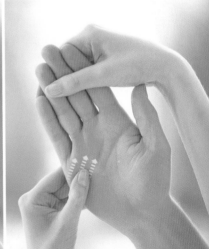

1 With your right thumb, make several passes over the HEART reflex area at the base of the thumb. Then starting at the DIAPHRAGM reflex area, repeatedly walk through the CHEST, LUNG and UPPER BACK reflex areas.

2 Move on to the next segment of the CHEST, LUNG and UPPER BACK reflex areas and apply the thumb-walking technique in a succession of passes.

3 Change hands. Hold the fingers back with the right hand and apply the thumb-walking technique with the left. Begin with the DIAPHRAGM reflex area and thumb walk up the SHOULDER reflex area.

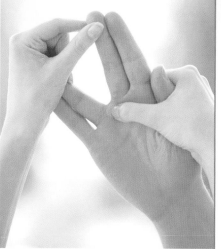

HAND ORIENTATION

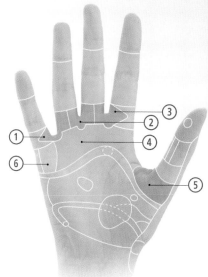

4 To work the EYE reflex area, spread and hold the index and middle fingers apart with the left hand. Position the thumb and index finger of your working hand to gently pinch the webbing between the fingers several times.

5 Position the thumb and index finger on the INNER EAR reflex area. Apply a gentle pinch to the webbing between the fingers several times.

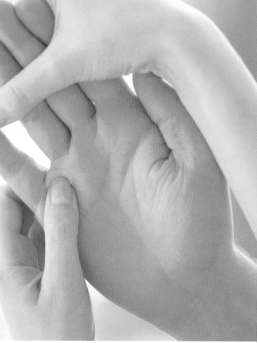

6 Change hands, moving on to the EAR reflex area. Pinch the webbing gently several times with the left thumb and index finger.

RIGHT HAND

Working the upper part of the palm targets three groups of reflex areas: the eyes and ears; the chest, lungs and heart; and the shoulders and upper back.

The EAR ①, INNER EAR ② and EYE ③ are located between the index and middle, middle and ring, and ring and little fingers respectively. The CHEST, LUNG, UPPER BACK reflex area is a band across the top of the palm ④. On the hand map these three areas occupy the same space but, in same way as the upper back is located behind the lungs, the upper back reflex area actually lies "behind" the lung and chest reflex areas. The HEART reflex area is located at the base of the thumb ⑤ and the SHOULDER at the base of the little finger ⑥.

The reflex areas on the left hand exactly mirror those on the right, with the left hand relating to the left side of the body and the right hand corresponding to the right.

DESSERTS   Palm-rocker (p. 100) • Hand-stretcher (p. 100) • Palm-mover (p. 101)

STEP 4

Working the centre and heel of the palm

This sequence primarily works reflex areas associated with the processing of food and the elimination of waste after digestion. The reflex areas worked here correspond to the liver, gall bladder, colon and small intestine. This part of the hand also includes the arm reflex area, which lies just below the little finger.

AREAS WORKED
LIVER & GALL BLADDER: Reflexology may help these organs regulate chemical levels in the blood, excreting the unwanted substances as bile.
ARMS: Prone to stiffness, these limbs may respond well to reflexology.
COLON: Apply reflexology to this area to aid in the storage and expulsion of waste products in the form of faecal matter.
SMALL INTESTINE: Working this reflex area may assist the small intestine in breaking down food.

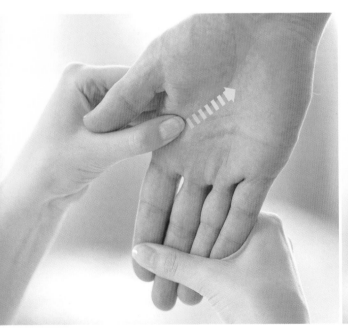

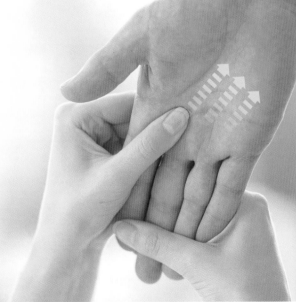

1 To work the LIVER and GALL BLADDER reflex areas, hold the hand in front of you with your right hand. Starting at the DIAPHRAGM reflex area, use your left thumb to apply the thumb-walking technique.

2 Now reposition the left thumb and continue thumb-walking with the left hand through the LIVER and GALL BLADDER reflex areas with a series of passes.

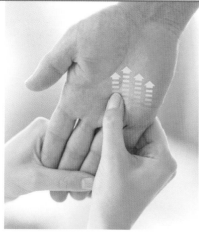 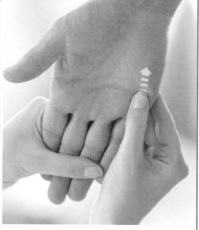

HAND ORIENTATION

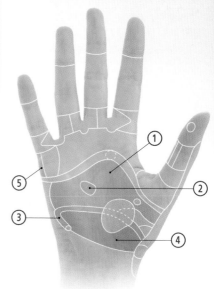

3 To continue work on the LIVER and GALL BLADDER reflex areas, change hands, holding the fingers with your left hand. Apply a series of thumb-walking passes with your right hand.

4 Next, position the right thumb and index finger to press on the fleshy outer part of the hand – the ARM reflex area. Reposition and press again, continuing up the hand.

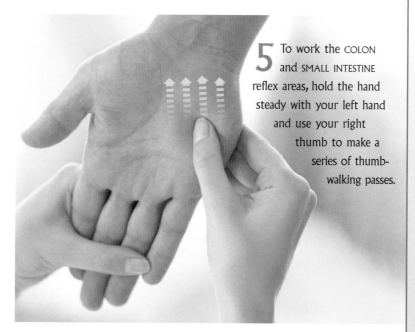

5 To work the COLON and SMALL INTESTINE reflex areas, hold the hand steady with your left hand and use your right thumb to make a series of thumb-walking passes.

DESSERTS   Finger-pull (p. 98) • Hand-stretcher (p. 100) • Palm-mover (p. 101)

RIGHT HAND

Working reflex areas in the fleshy parts of the palm and the heel of the hand mostly targets reflex areas relating to the digestive organs.

The large LIVER area stretches across the palm (1), enclosing the GALL BLADDER reflex area (2). The COLON reflex area runs across the heel of the hand (3) bordering the SMALL INTESTINE area (4). The ARM reflex area is located in the fleshy pad just below the little finger (5).

Usually the reflex areas on the left and right hands mirror one another exactly. However, the gall bladder and the liver reflex areas feature only on the right hand, and not on the left. On the left hand the spleen lies in a position approximately corresponding to that of the gall bladder on the right hand. The different parts of the colon are reflected on the hands in the same way they are on the feet (see page 83).

STEP 5

Working the tops of the fingers and the side of the thumb

This sequence should not only help to relax muscular tension in the spine, but also relieve any associated pain. Work the spinal reflex area on the side of the thumb, and the other reflex areas found on the tops of the fingers and the thumb to treat the spine, head, sinuses, neck, teeth, gums and jaw.

1 To work the SPINE, hold the hand upright with your left hand. Start with the TAILBONE reflex area and use your right thumb to walk up along the bony edge of the hand. Continue up through the midback area of the SPINE reflex area, too. Make several passes.

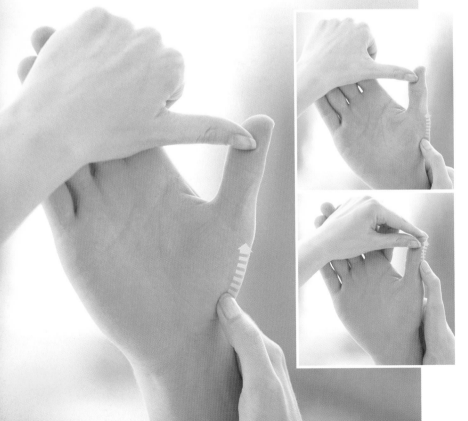

2 To continue working the SPINE, hold the thumb steady with your left hand. Walk your right thumb through the UPPER BACK reflex area.

3 Continue by thumb-walking with the right hand through the NECK reflex area.

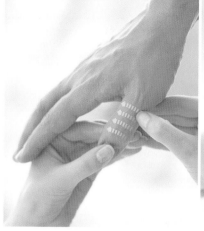

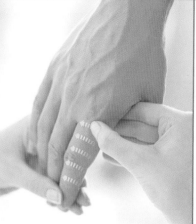

HAND ORIENTATION

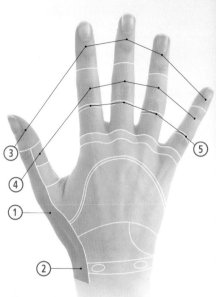

4 To work the HEAD, BRAIN, SINUS, NECK, TEETH, GUMS and JAW reflex areas, begin by holding the thumb steady with your left hand. Thumb-walk with your right hand across the top of the thumb several times.

5 Move on to the index finger, to work the next portion of these reflex areas. Hold the finger in place with the left hand and thumb-walk through the area with the right thumb. Repeat several times.

RIGHT HAND

Working the tops of the fingers and the side of the thumb targets the spine and anatomical structures of the face and head.

Replicating the way the spine runs down the back, the reflex area for the SPINE runs down the inside of the thumb (1), with the TAILBONE area at the bottom, near the wrist (2). The areas representing the HEAD, BRAIN and SINUS all occupy the same reflex area, which runs from the tip to the first joint on each of the five digits (3). Underneath it – again on each of the five digits – is the reflex area for the NECK (4). Finally the reflex area for the TEETH, GUMS and the JAW is a very narrow band at the second joint on each finger (5).

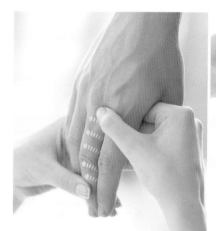

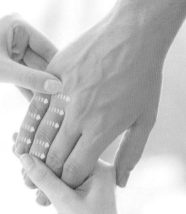

6 On the middle finger, work the next portion of the HEAD, BRAIN, SINUS, NECK, TEETH, GUMS and JAW reflex areas. Steady the finger and thumb-walk through the area.

7 Change hands to work the HEAD, BRAIN, SINUS, NECK, TEETH, GUMS and JAW reflex areas thoroughly on the ring finger, before repeating the sequence on the little finger.

The reflex areas on the right and left hand mirror one another perfectly, with the left hand relating to areas on the left side of the body, and the right hand relating to the right side of the body.

DESSERTS   Palm-rocker (p. 100) • Hand-stretcher (p. 100) • Palm-mover (p. 101)

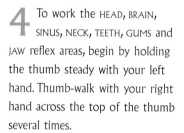

STEP 6
Working the top of the hand

This sequence works reflex areas corresponding to respiration, milk production, heart action and the musculo-skeletal structure of the upper body. The reflex areas on the top of the right hand correspond to parts of the right side of the body: lung, chest, breast, lower back, lymph glands, groin, knee, leg and ovary or testicle. Work these locations to stimulate and enhance function in these areas of the body.

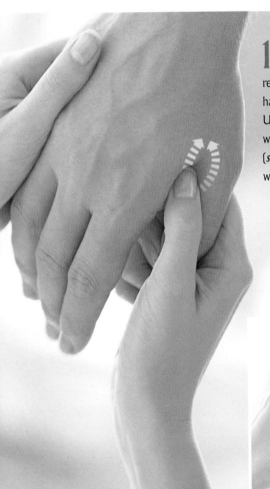

1 To work the LUNG, CHEST, BREAST and UPPER BACK reflex areas, first steady the hand with your left hand. Use the right thumb to walk down the long bone (*see page 41*) at the side of the webbing of the hand. Repeat.

AREAS WORKED

CHEST & LUNGS: Apply techniques to these reflex areas to help to loosen a tight chest and open up passageways in the lungs.

BREAST: Use reflexology to help regulate the production of milk in lactating women.

UPPER & LOWER BACK: Working these reflex areas may ease pain in the back.

LYMPH GLANDS, FALLOPIAN TUBES & GROIN: These areas may respond well to reflexology.

OVARIES/TESTICLES: To enhance function of the female and male sex organs, use reflexology techniques regularly.

UTERUS/PROSTATE GLAND: The application of reflexology work aims to enhance function of the uterus in females and prostate gland in males.

2 To work the next part of these reflex areas, change hands. The right hand holds the hand steady while the left thumb walks between the long bones, making a series of passes up the top of the hand.

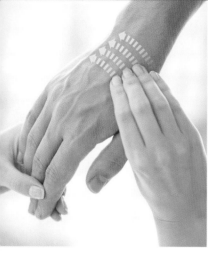

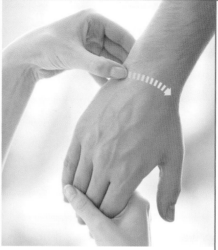

3 Next, use all four fingers on the right hand to finger-walk across the LOWER BACK reflex area. Repeat several times.

4 Change hands and walk the left thumb through the LYMPH GLANDS, FALLOPIAN TUBES and GROIN reflex areas. Make a series of passes.

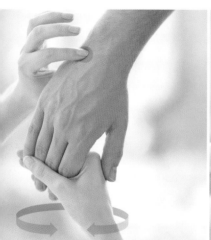

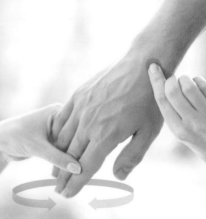

5 Pinpoint the OVARY/TESTICLE reflex area with your left index finger. Use the rotating on a point technique, moving the hand in a clockwise direction, then anti-clockwise. Repeat.

6 Change hands and pinpoint the UTERUS/PROSTATE GLAND reflex area, rotating the hand repeatedly in a clockwise direction and then in an anti-clockwise direction.

DESSERTS   Finger-pull (p. 98) • Hand-stretcher (p. 100) • Palm-mover (p. 101)

HAND ORIENTATION

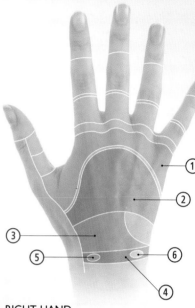

RIGHT HAND

The back of the hand contains reflex areas in wide bands. Close to the fingers is the reflex area for the UPPER BACK, LUNG, CHEST and BREAST ①. Though drawn as one area, the upper back reflex area lies on top of the others – mirroring the way that on the body the back is on the surface with the lungs "beneath" it. There is a second reflex area for the upper back ② and, moving towards the wrist, the LOWER BACK reflex area ③.

In a narrow band near the wrist is the reflex area for the LYMPH GLANDS, FALLOPIAN TUBES and GROIN ④. Within this, the reflex area for the TESTICLE in men or the OVARY in women can be found ⑤, and also the area for the PROSTATE GLAND (in men) and the UTERUS (in women) ⑥.

The left hand exactly mirrors the right hand, and reflex areas on the right hand correspond to the right side of the body, while reflex areas on the left hand relate to the left.

STEP 7
Working the left hand

Once you have worked through the full sequence on the right hand, it's time to move on to the left hand. These pages outline the sequence for a left-hand workout, and also provide a useful workout summary. Once you've become familiar with how techniques are applied to each part of the hand, this summary provides an at-a-glance reminder of the complete sequence.

DESSERTS

Before beginning the sequence, check the hand cuts, bruises and areas to b avoided when working

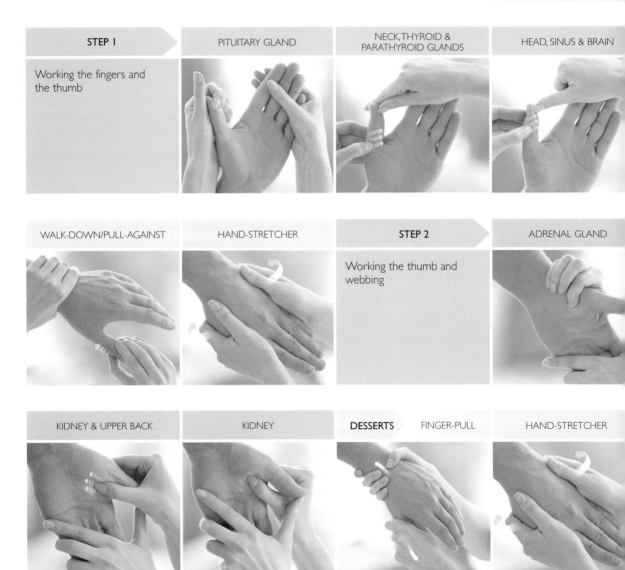

STEP 1	PITUITARY GLAND	NECK, THYROID & PARATHYROID GLANDS	HEAD, SINUS & BRAIN
Working the fingers and the thumb			

WALK-DOWN/PULL-AGAINST	HAND-STRETCHER	STEP 2	ADRENAL GLAND
		Working the thumb and webbing	

KIDNEY & UPPER BACK	KIDNEY	DESSERTS FINGER-PULL	HAND-STRETCHER

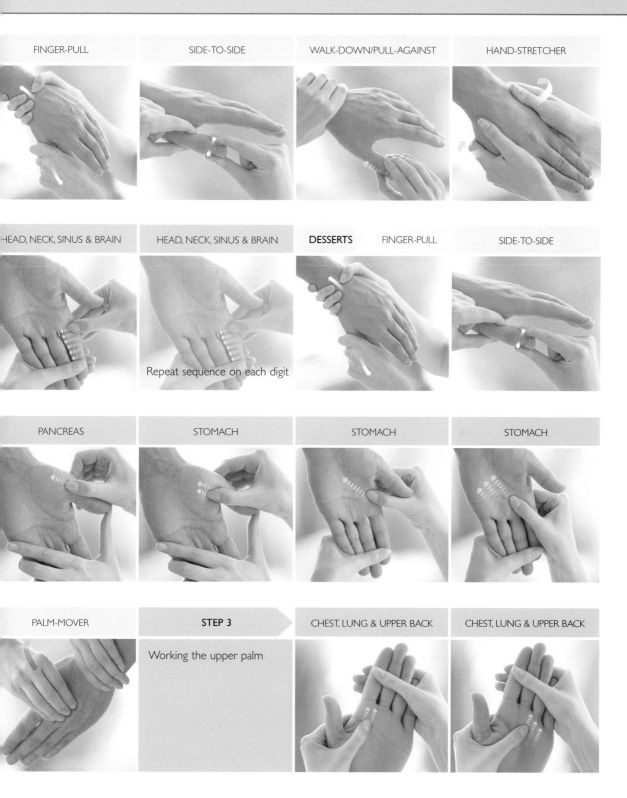

FINGER-PULL	SIDE-TO-SIDE	WALK-DOWN/PULL-AGAINST	HAND-STRETCHER

HEAD, NECK, SINUS & BRAIN	HEAD, NECK, SINUS & BRAIN	DESSERTS FINGER-PULL	SIDE-TO-SIDE

Repeat sequence on each digit

PANCREAS	STOMACH	STOMACH	STOMACH

PALM-MOVER	STEP 3	CHEST, LUNG & UPPER BACK	CHEST, LUNG & UPPER BACK

Working the upper palm

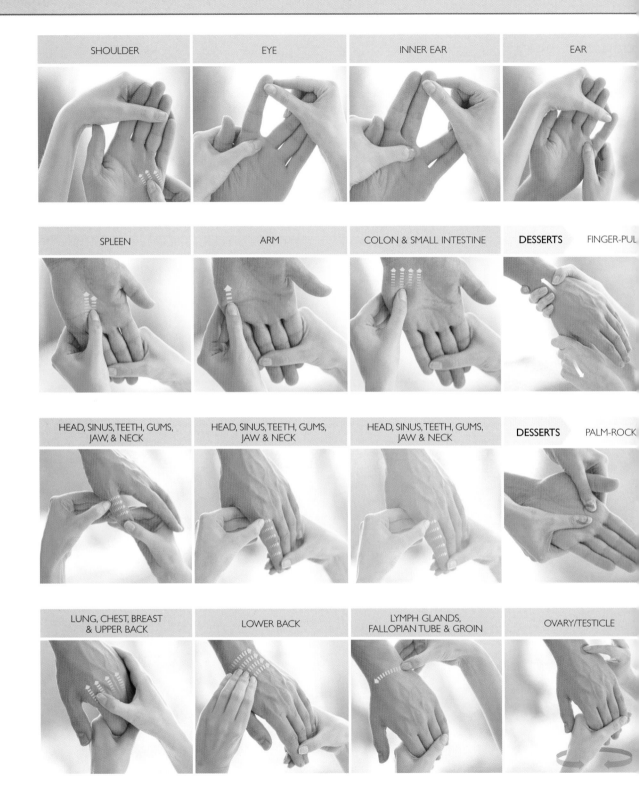

SHOULDER	EYE	INNER EAR	EAR

SPLEEN	ARM	COLON & SMALL INTESTINE	**DESSERTS** FINGER-PUL

HEAD, SINUS, TEETH, GUMS, JAW, & NECK	HEAD, SINUS, TEETH, GUMS, JAW & NECK	HEAD, SINUS, TEETH, GUMS, JAW & NECK	**DESSERTS** PALM-ROCK

LUNG, CHEST, BREAST & UPPER BACK	LOWER BACK	LYMPH GLANDS, FALLOPIAN TUBE & GROIN	OVARY/TESTICLE

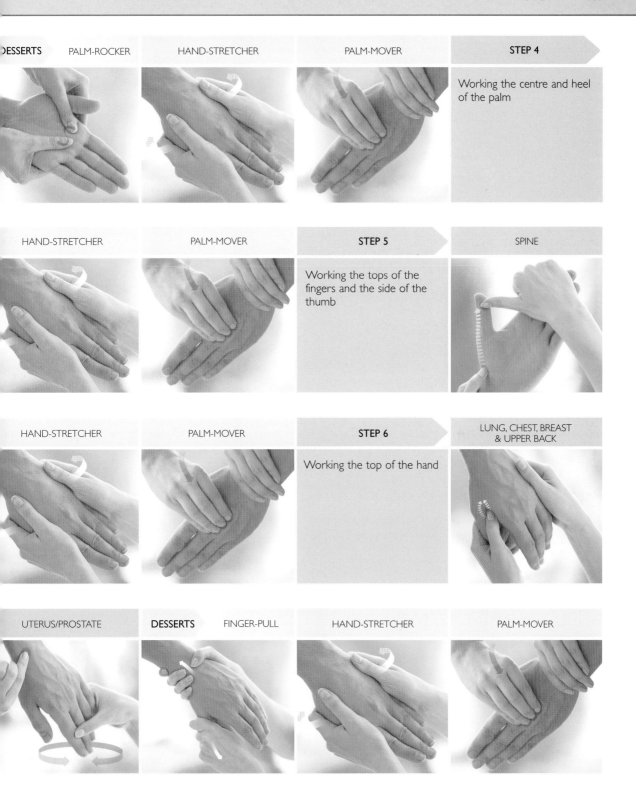

DESSERTS   PALM-ROCKER

HAND-STRETCHER

PALM-MOVER

STEP 4

Working the centre and heel of the palm

HAND-STRETCHER

PALM-MOVER

STEP 5

Working the tops of the fingers and the side of the thumb

SPINE

HAND-STRETCHER

PALM-MOVER

STEP 6

Working the top of the hand

LUNG, CHEST, BREAST & UPPER BACK

UTERUS/PROSTATE

DESSERTS   FINGER-PULL

HAND-STRETCHER

PALM-MOVER

PEOPLE WITH SPECIFIC NEEDS

Certain groups of people require extra consideration in reflexology work. Sequences need to be adapted, for instance, to suit babies, children, pregnant women and the elderly. In general, start gradually: increase the duration of the workout and the strength of your pressure over the course of several workouts. At the end of the session, work the kidney reflex areas to encourage elimination of toxins.

Babies

A little reflexology goes a long way with babies. Gentle touch is all that is needed to work tiny feet and hands. Concerns often include sleep, colic and diarrhoea.

POINTS TO REMEMBER
Be gentle.
Work briefly with one or two reflex areas.
To work further, gently press parts of the hand and foot.

Children

Reflexology work with children establishes a bond, creates a quiet time together, helps relaxation and lets you find the "silent owies" – those falls and bumps that young ones don't always mention. The following workout targets reflex areas of concern for children. Work through the reflex areas indicated first on the right foot and then on the left, or work the corresponding hand reflex areas instead.

POINTS TO REMEMBER
Don't expect to apply a full workout to a young child. Attention spans are short at this age.
Make a game of it. For example, play "This little piggy went to market" while working with the toes.
Monkey see, monkey do: if you apply self-help techniques, your child will too.
Keep your touch light. A child who withdraws a foot from you is telling you something.

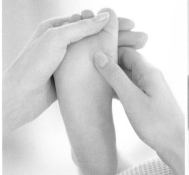

1 Holding the foot steady, gently press the SOLAR PLEXUS area with the thumb of your working hand. This step is designed to relieve any tension in the child.

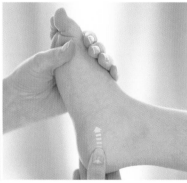

2 Next, thumb-walk up the TAILBONE reflex area, passing over the area several times to counter the impact of falls frequently experienced by children.

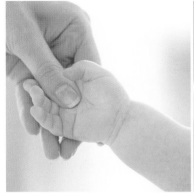 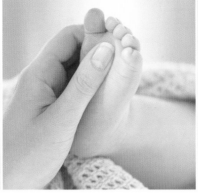 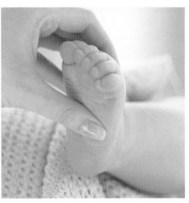

1 To calm a baby, gently press your thumb on the SOLAR PLEXUS reflex area in the webbing of the hand. Repeat this on the baby's other hand.

2 Using your thumb, lightly press the OESOPHAGUS reflex area, located in the ball of the foot, to ease colic. Repeat on other foot.

3 Gently press your thumb on the COLON reflex area to treat diarrhoea. Now repeat on the other foot.

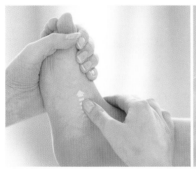 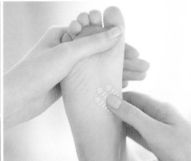 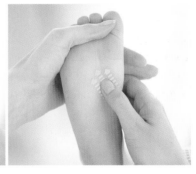

3 Continue thumb-walking up the SPINE reflex area several times to further counter injuries.

4 Then thumb-walk repeatedly through the PANCREAS reflex area to help regulate these glands.

5 Next, thumb-walk through the ADRENAL GLAND reflex area to continue the focus on the glands.

6 Work the UTERUS/ PROSTATE GLAND reflex area, applying the rotating-on-a-point technique, to enhance function.

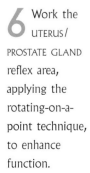 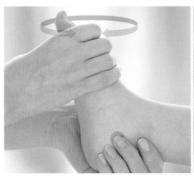 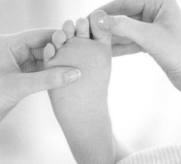

7 Then hook and back-up repeatedly through the PITUITARY GLAND reflex area to stimulate the body's "master gland".

Pregnant women

Concerns of pregnant women vary from time to time. Establish a goal for your workout. Adjust your session to address the need for relaxation, relieving an aching lower back or swollen feet / hands / body; or combine all the techniques to address several needs. Apply techniques to the reflex areas indicated on the right foot, and then go on to work the left. Shown here are foot sequences, but you could equally well work the corresponding hand reflex areas instead if you prefer.

CAUTION

Whether or not it is safe to apply reflexology work to pregnant women in the first trimester is a matter of debate within the profession. Our view is that reflexology work is beneficial if you:

• Start gradually, working for a short time and with a light touch.

• Avoid applying repeated work to one reflex area for an extended period of time.
• Do apply work to the kidney reflex area.
• Encourage consultation with a doctor if any irregularities appear.

---

2 Apply the SIDE-TO-SIDE dessert for general relaxation.

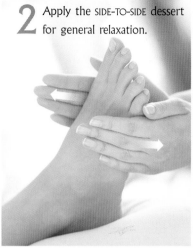

3 Next, use the SOLE-MOVER dessert to further enhance relaxation.

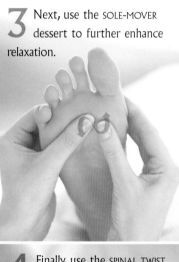

4 Finally, use the SPINAL TWIST dessert to ease any tension in the spinal column.

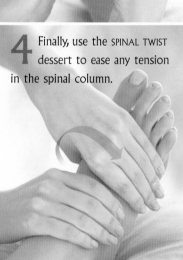

To promote general relaxation

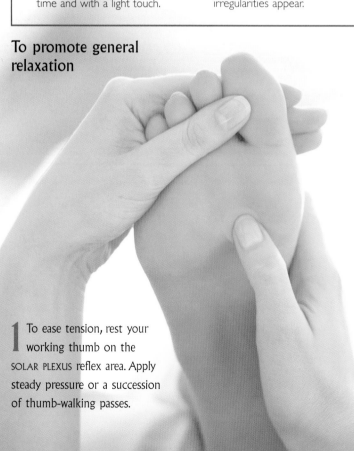

1 To ease tension, rest your working thumb on the SOLAR PLEXUS reflex area. Apply steady pressure or a succession of thumb-walking passes.

To soothe an aching lower back

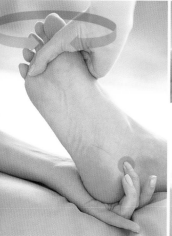 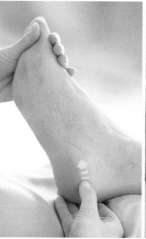 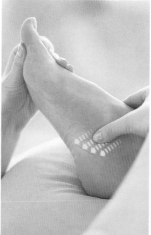 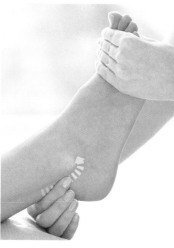

1 Apply the rotating-on-a-point technique to the UTERUS reflex area to relieve any related tension.

2 Next, thumb-walk repeatedly up the TAILBONE reflex area to work the sacral vertebrae.

3 Work the BLADDER and LOWER BACK reflex areas thoroughly to relax and relieve them.

4 Finally, finger-walk along the HIP and SCIATIC NERVE reflex areas to work them thoroughly.

To relieve swelling

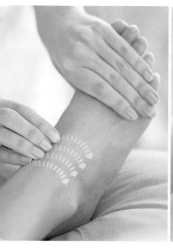 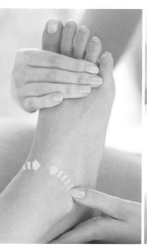 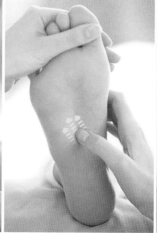 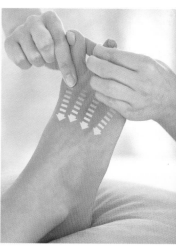

1 Finger-walk across the LOWER BACK reflex area with all four fingers to stimulate swollen areas.

2 Thumb-walk through the LYMPH GLAND reflex area to encourage lymph drainage.

3 Work the KIDNEY reflex area to promote elimination of waste fluids.

4 Finger-walk down the BREAST and CHEST reflex areas to encourage upper lymph drainage.

Elderly people

The aspect of reflexology many older people most often enjoy is the addition of touch to their day, and a relaxing session can improve their quality of life. The elderly have special concerns that can be addressed though reflexology, including restricted movement, incontinence and aching joints (*see also Arthritis & Rheumatism, page 142*). The workouts shown here target each concern or can be combined for multiple ailments. Apply the following techniques to the reflex areas indicated on the right foot, then on the left. These are foot sequences, but alternatively you could work the same reflex areas on the hands if you wish.

To encourage joint flexibility

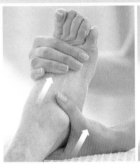

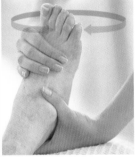

1 First, apply gentle ANKLE TRACTION to "loosen up" the bones of the foot.

2 Next, use the ANKLE ROTATION dessert to work the ankle through its full range of movement.

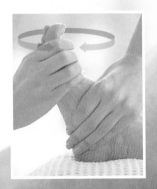

3 Use the MID-FOOT MOVER to promote general "loosening up" and flexibility in the foot.

4 Follow this with the SIDE-TO-SIDE dessert to relax the foot in general.

To treat incontinence

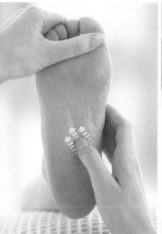
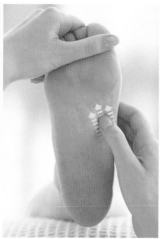
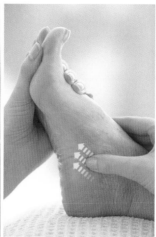
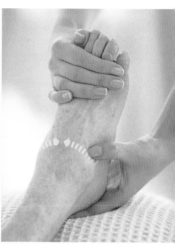

1 Thumb-walk through the KIDNEY reflex area repeatedly to stimulate these organs.

2 Next, thumb-walk several times through the reflex area for the ADRENAL GLAND to encourage muscle tone.

3 Move round to work the BLADDER reflex area thoroughly to stimulate urine production.

4 Finally, thumb-walk through the LYMPH GLAND reflex area to help ease fluid retention.

To relieve aching joints

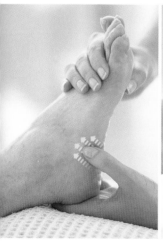
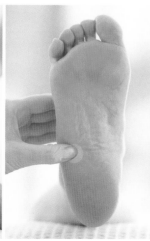
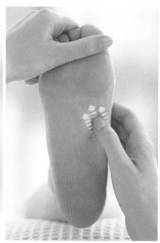
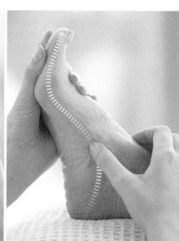

1 Work the KNEE and LEG reflex areas several times to ease any associated pain.

2 Then, hook and back-up several times through the COLON reflex area to help facilitate mobility.

3 Thumb-walk through the ADRENAL GLAND reflex area thoroughly to aid in calming inflammation.

4 End by repeatedly thumb-walking up through the SPINE reflex area to relax the vertebrae.

SELF-HELP

Performing reflexology on yourself has several advantages, such as convenience. You can also judge how a certain reflex zone feels and then decide which areas are most sensitive or in need of more work. The reflex areas selected here address general health. To target a more specific health concern, however, see pages 130–53.

Self-help for the feet

These movements aim to relax the foot and encourage movement seldom experienced during the day. If you have difficulty reaching your feet, try the self-help sequence on the hands (*see page 126*) instead.

Self-help foot desserts

First, apply a series of desserts, such as the ones listed below. These exercises will promote relaxation and break up the stress patterns formed during the course of an average day.

LEARNING TIPS

If you find it difficult to reach your feet to apply techniques, consider using hand reflexology techniques, or a foot roller or stroll path.

Create "found" time in a busy schedule by applying technique while doing something else or by simply finding a few minutes here and there for light reflexology work.

Get results and get motivated. Pick a small area to begin with. Decide on a health concern and apply the appropriate techniques.

Experiment with various techniques to find the one(s) that you like and therefore will apply often enough to get results.

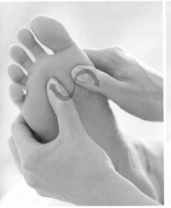
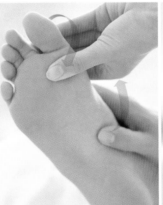
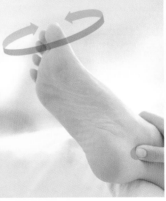
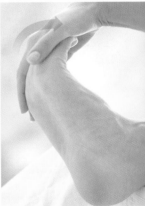

1 First apply the SOLE-MOVER dessert technique to relax the LUNG reflex area in the ball of the foot (*see page 71 for instructions*).

2 Relax the spinal reflex area by applying the SPINAL TWIST dessert technique (*see page 69 for instructions*).

3 Finally, apply the ANKLE ROTATION dessert, which not only relaxes the four major muscle groups in the foot, but also helps to relieve water retention round the ankles (*see page 72 for instructions*).

4 To encourage relaxation in the neck and upper back, stretch the sole of the foot (*see above*).

Self-help foot sequence

After applying a series of desserts, follow the steps in this self-help sequence for a simple, general foot reflexology workout.

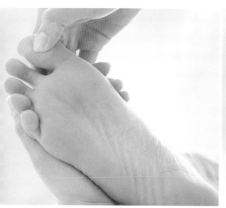

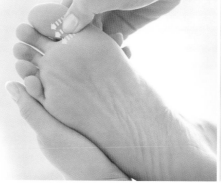

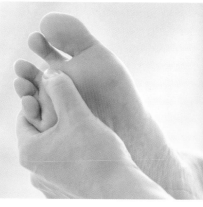

1 Rest your foot on your other leg. Hook and back up several times through the PITUITARY GLAND reflex area, supporting your foot with your holding hand.

2 Move on to the NECK, THYROID and PARATHYROID GLAND reflex areas. Supporting the foot with your holding hand, use your other thumb to "walk" several passes through the reflex areas.

3 Next, pinch several times between the toes with the tip of the thumb to work the reflex areas for the EYE, INNER EAR and EAR respectively.

4 Press your thumb on the reflex area for the UTERUS/PROSTATE GLAND. Rotate your foot clockwise and then anti-clockwise several times. Try to draw 360° circles with your big toe.

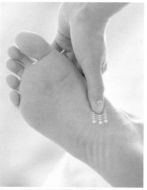

5 To work the PANCREAS reflex area, thumb-walk towards the inside of the foot at the waistline. Make several successive passes.

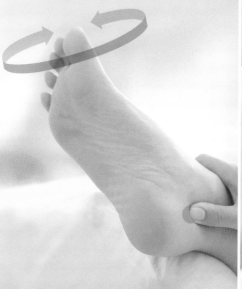

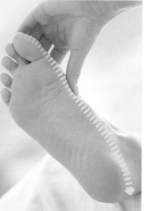

6 To work the SPINE reflex area, place your fingers round the big toe and rest your thumb on the inside of the foot. Thumb-walk down the inside edge of the foot. When your thumb feels stretched, reposition it and walk down a further portion of the reflex area.

Self-help for the hands

Your hands are ideal for a discreet self-help workout. You might also keep a golf ball within reach – by your chair, in your handbag or at your desk for a quick stress break. Begin with a series of desserts to relax and prepare the hand. (*To address specific ailments, see pages 130–53.*)

Self-help hand desserts

The desserts listed below can be applied before embarking on the self-help hand sequence. You could also supplement these with the other hand desserts (*see pages 98–101*), to further relax the hands.

1 Pull gently on your finger, turning your hand from side to side gently. Repeat and apply the FINGER-PULL technique to each of the other fingers.

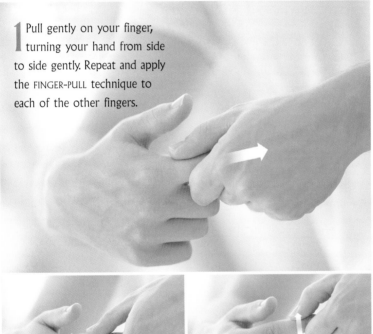

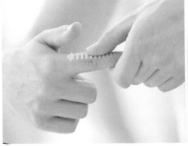

2 Next, apply the WALK-DOWN/ PULL-AGAINST technique to stretch the joints comfortably, making several passes along each digit (*see page 99 for instructions*).

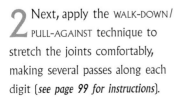

3 The FINGER SIDE-TO-SIDE dessert will help move the fingers in a way that provides a contrast with their usual usage patterns. Repeat several times on each digit (*see page 99 for instructions*).

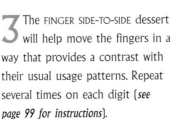

Self-help hand sequence

After applying a series of hand desserts, work a variety of reflex

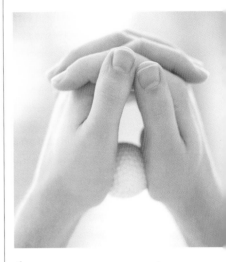

1 To work the PANCREAS and STOMACH reflex areas, rest a golf ball between your hands and roll it throughout the areas, or thumb-walk several times through the areas.

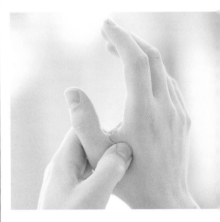

5 Rest your thumb and fingertip in the SOLAR PLEXUS area, in the webbing of the hand. Pinch the thumb and fingertip together several times.

areas with the following steps. This self-help sequence targets commonly stressed reflex areas. Some techniques use a self-help tool, such as the golf ball used here, or a purpose-made reflexology tool.

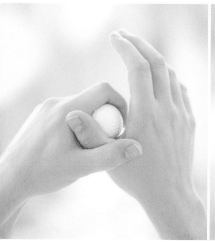

2 Now grasp the golf ball and rest it on the THYROID GLAND reflex area. Roll it back and forth several times.

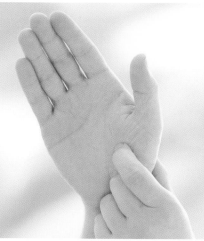

3 Rest your fingertip on the ADRENAL GLAND reflex area (*see page 104 for hints on locating the adrenal gland reflex area*). Alternate pressure, repeating several times.

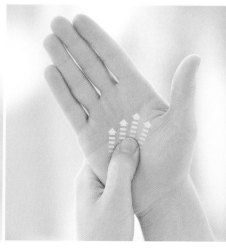

4 To work the LIVER and GALL BLADDER reflex areas, position your thumb in the palm of the hand. Use the thumb-walking technique to walk through the areas.

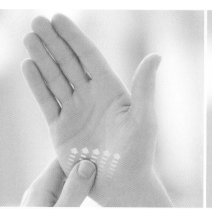

6 Move on to work the COLON and SMALL INTESTINE reflex areas, thumb-walking repeatedly through these areas in the heel of the hand.

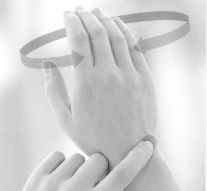

7 Place your index finger on the OVARY / TESTICLE area of the other hand, located on your wrist. Now use the rotating on a point technique (*see page 66 for instructions*) several times in both directions.

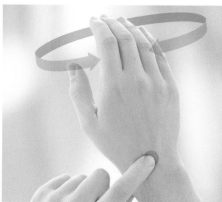

8 Now reposition the same finger on the UTERUS / PROSTATE GLAND reflex areas, also on the wrist. Repeatedly apply the rotating-on-a-point technique, first in a clockwise and then anti-clockwise direction.

Reflexology for the office

There's nothing like feeling under par to make a work day seem longer. Your reflexology skills can help you improve the day. The reflex areas noted here are aimed at boosting your energy levels and helping you cope with stress. If your hands are tired from the work they've done, try the exercises on page 54.

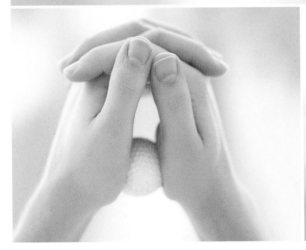

Hand rocks back and forth to create "on/off" pressure

1 First, place your fingertip on the ADRENAL GLAND reflex area and apply pressure. Now rock your working hand from side to side. Change hands and repeat the sequence on the other hand. This energising movement will prepare you for a busy day.

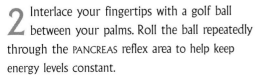

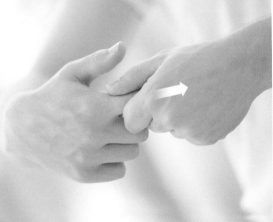

2 Interlace your fingertips with a golf ball between your palms. Roll the ball repeatedly through the PANCREAS reflex area to help keep energy levels constant.

3 To round out this sequence, relieve office-related tension and revive overworked hands, finish with the application of the FINGER-PULL dessert. Repeat on each finger. Repeat the sequence on the other hand.

Reflexology on the move

Transform commuting time into time found for improving health. By subtly applying reflexology techniques, you can prepare yourself for the busy day or wind down for a relaxed evening. Try the following exercises for common commuter concerns, or target specific health concerns (*see pages 130–53*).

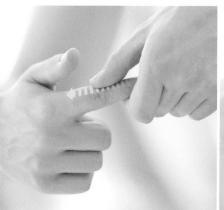 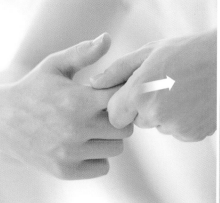 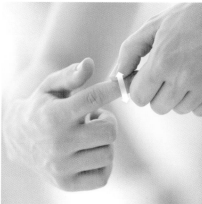

1 This movement relaxes the NECK area and gently stretches the fingers of sore commuter hands. Use the WALK-DOWN/PULL-AGAINST technique along each finger of both hands in succession.

2 Apply the FINGER-PULL dessert to relax the fingers. Repeat on each finger. Now change hands and repeat the sequence on the other hand.

3 The FINGER SIDE-TO-SIDE promotes flexibility in the fingers and gives them a break from their usual patterns of movement. Repeat on each finger of one hand, then change hands and repeat the sequence on the other hand.

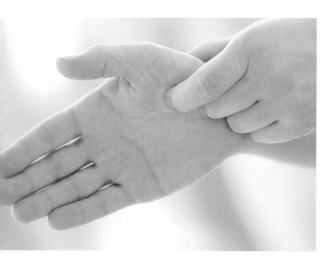 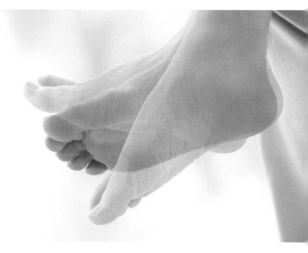

4 Apply pressure to the ADRENAL GLAND reflex area to ready yourself for the morning rush hour. Using your index fingertip, rock your working hand from side to side. Repeat this movement on the other hand.

5 Use the ANKLE ROTATION technique to stretch foot muscles and to soothe sore commuter feet. Rotate your foot several times clockwise and then several times in an anti-clockwise direction. Change legs and repeat.

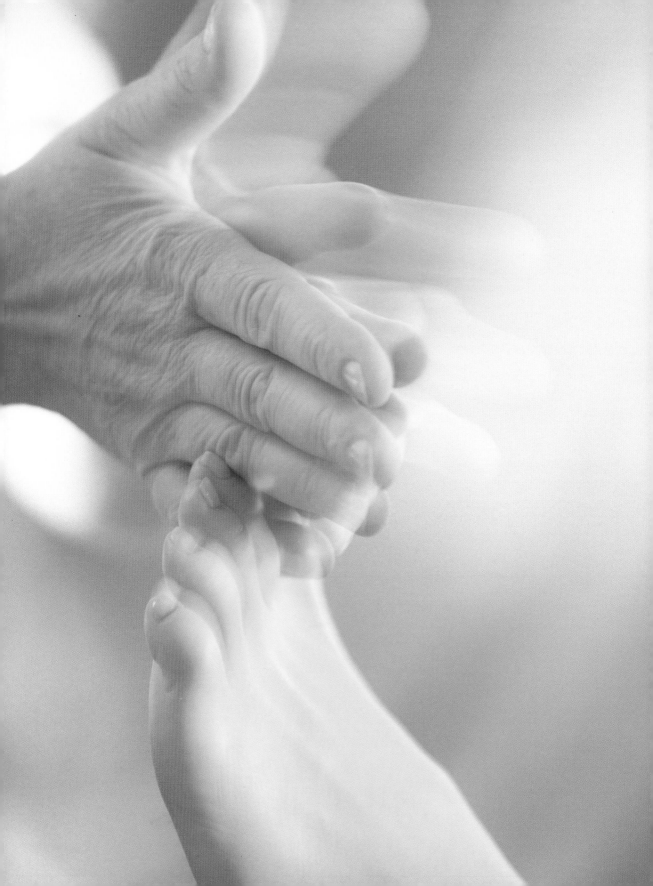

REFLEXOLOGY TO TARGET HEALTH CONCERNS

Whether you want to soothe a sore throat, help

ease an asthma attack or relieve a headache,

reflexology is a safe and convenient adjunct to

conventional medical treatment. In addition to the

in-depth pages on selected disorders, this chapter

also includes a quick-reference chart listing relevant

reflex areas to work for a wide range of health

concerns. For each ailment, you're given a couple of

reflex areas to target on both your hands and feet.

USING REFLEXOLOGY FOR HEALTH CONCERNS

While the reflexology sequences shown earlier in this book concern the whole foot and hand and aim to improve general health and well-being, you can also work specific reflex areas to help target particular health concerns. You can target reflex areas for health concerns following a full reflexology workout or, if you have less time or want to focus solely on a particular health concern, you can just apply reflexology techniques to specific reflex areas. In this section, we explain which reflex areas to work and how often to work them in order to encourage the body's natural self-healing powers. Many people find that working the feet has a more powerful effect than working the hands, but working the latter is often more convenient. Throughout we have specified reflex areas for both.

It is sometimes self-evident which reflex areas should be worked. For example, one applies reflexology work to the lung reflex area to have an impact on the function of the lungs. It makes sense, therefore, to target the lung reflex areas for bronchitis, asthma and other respiratory conditions.

Reflexologists have discovered over the years, however, that many factors can have an impact on health concerns and, therefore, that a variety of reflex areas need to be worked. For example, as well as working the lung reflex area, working the adrenal gland reflex area may help to relieve the symptoms of asthma. This is because targeting this reflex area helps to enhance the body's natural self-healing mechanisms. The adrenal glands are responsible for manufacturing adrenaline, which has an important role in helping the lungs to function well. Work applied to the adrenal gland reflex areas, therefore, may help to reduce wheezing and other symptoms of asthma.

In addition, many health concerns result from multiple factors. Constipation, for example, can result from tension and/or the malfunctioning of any one of the different organs that contribute to digestion

and elimination. To have an impact on constipation, reflexologists will work the stomach, colon and other reflex areas to get the desired result. When you apply reflexology to target health concerns, be prepared to experiment and take note of which seems to be the best reflex areas to work.

There are no precise rules on how long and how often you should apply reflexology technique work to particular reflex areas. To some extent it depends on the nature of the health concern and the age and general health of the person on whom you are working (*see Cautions, right*). Sometimes, you will want to work a reflex area continuously until you achieve the result you're seeking. An example of a case such as this might be finding relief from an uncomfortable menstrual period. If the health concern you are addressing is persistent and has existed for a number of years, for example, if you regularly have constipation or headaches, you will want to work the appropriate reflex areas every day and perhaps 3–4 times a day. Listen to your body and take note of how long and how often you need to work the reflex areas to get relief from the problem.

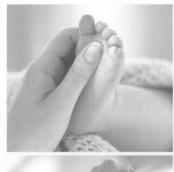

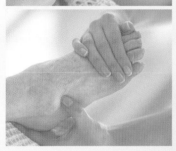

CAUTIONS

- Reflexology is an adjunct to medical care, not a substitute. Always consult your doctor if you have a medical condition.
- If pregnant, be aware of the specific cautions that apply (see page 120).
- If you work with children, babies, or the elderly, work more frequently, but with less pressure and for a shorter period of time than when working with adults (see also pages 118–23).
- If a reflex area becomes very sensitive to touch, it has been over-worked, so work elsewhere. When you once again work the area on another day, work it more frequently but use less pressure and work it only for a short period of time.
- When working with the pancreas reflex area of individuals with diabetes or hypoglycaemia (low blood sugar), work only lightly and briefly to begin with.
- Do not overwork a reflex area that reflects an infected body part, e.g. the bladder reflex area for a bladder infection concern.
- When working with someone who is severely ill, work only for brief periods of time, applying light pressure.

TIPS FOR ADDRESSING HEALTH CONCERNS

TENSION RELIEF: Stress and tension contribute to many health concerns. Reflexology offers three strategies for relieving tension.

1. Apply a full foot or hand reflexology sequence. On the whole, a reflexology workout from someone else is more relaxing than working on yourself.
2. Consider a "dessert workout," applying dessert after dessert (see pages 68–73 and 98–101).
3. Work the solar plexus reflex area, applying a lengthy series of passes at the beginning and end of your workout.

FEEL-GOOD RESPONSE: During reflexology work, it's common for someone to say "That feels good" or even "That hurts good". Take note of the reflex area or dessert they are referring to for future work.

WORK WITHIN THE COMFORT ZONE: A comment of "That hurts" or a foot or hand being drawn away indicates that a reflex area is very sensitive or the pressure is too strong. Always work within the individual's comfort zone.

PLENTY OF WATER: Always remind people to drink plenty of water to rid the body of toxins following reflexology work.

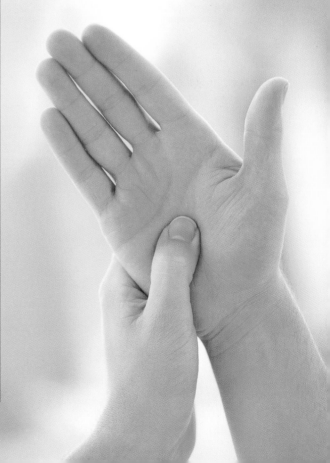

CONSTIPATION

Constipation, which is the sluggish action of the bowels, may often respond well to reflexology work. Many factors can adversely affect the elimination process, including diet, lack of water, certain medications and injury to the lower back. Working reflex areas that correspond to the digestive tract may help bring relief.

Working the hands

The reflex areas for the digestive organs are found on both hands and cover a wide area. Using a golf ball allows you to cover these broad reflex areas easily, working both hands at once.

1 Roll the golf ball along the heel of the hand below the thumb to work the ADRENAL GLANDS and part of the PANCREAS and STOMACH areas.

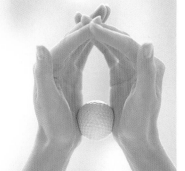

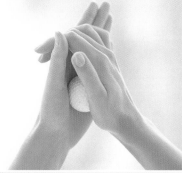

2 Now reposition the golf ball between the heels of your hands. Roll it over the COLON and SMALL INTESTINE reflex areas.

3 Move on, holding the golf ball in position to roll through the STOMACH reflex area on the left hand.

4 Change hands and roll the ball through the GALL BLADDER and LIVER reflex areas on the right hand.

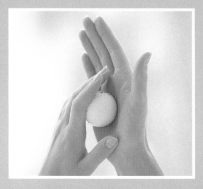

Working the feet

When applying reflexology to the feet for constipation, work the reflex areas corresponding to digestion and elimination. First work the right foot evenly, then repeat the sequence on the left. Take note of how long you work reflex areas and what results you achieve for future reference.

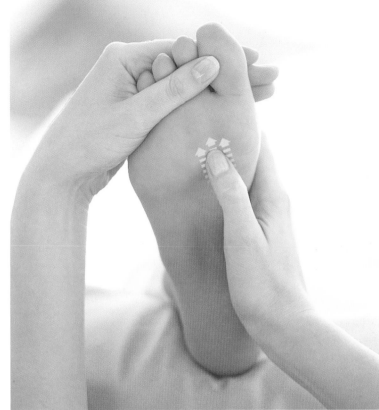

1 Begin by applying a series of thumb-walking passes to the SOLAR PLEXUS reflex area. This can help to relieve tension, which often contributes to constipation.

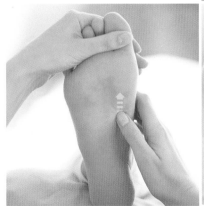

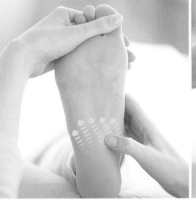

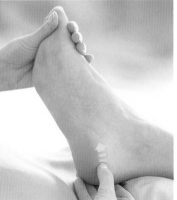

2 Thumb-walk through the ADRENAL GLAND reflex area, making repeated passes. The action of the adrenal glands is essential to peristalsis (wave-like contractions of the small intestine and colon which propel food along).

3 Now work the GALL BLADDER, LIVER, COLON and SMALL INTESTINE reflex areas. Thumb-walk first from one direction and then from the other. The liver and gall bladder produce and store bile needed for digestion.

4 Finally, thumb-walk through the TAILBONE and RECTUM reflex areas, making repeated passes, to ease tension in the lower back. The colon and small intestine are enclosed by the pelvis and lower spine and any tension here can affect digestion.

HEADACHES

There are many factors which can contribute to a headache, but tension is nearly always a culprit. To most successfully deal with a headache, experiment with the sequences below and then apply reflexology techniques to the appropriate reflex areas (*see chart opposite*), depending on whether you have a migraine or whether the pain is in a particular part of your head.

<table>
<tr><td>RESEARCH</td></tr>
<tr><td>A Danish study in 1997 found that reflexology helped ease headaches. Most importantly, many participants came to think of "working on" their headaches rather than just "living with" them. The study concluded: "The patients see themselves as vital agents in the process of illness and of curing themselves."</td></tr>
</table>

Working the hands

Hand reflexology has many advantages. You can work your hands discreetly even in an office or other public place. Reflexes on the digits correspond to the head and neck, providing an easily accessible target area. Neck tension frequently contributes to headaches, and working the neck reflex areas may relieve this. Remember to work both hands evenly, experimenting to see what works best for you.

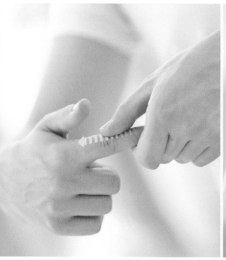

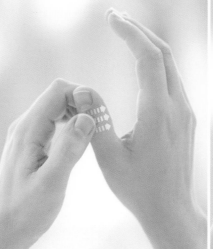

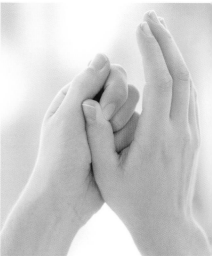

1 First, work the NECK and HEAD reflex areas to relieve tension using the walk-down/ pull-against dessert (*see page 99*). Try to visualise your neck and head stretching as you stretch the fingers.

2 Work the HEAD, FACE and SINUS reflex areas of the digits, focusing on tender areas. Work the areas just below the nails, seeking out sensitive spots. Depending on where the headache is located, you may get better results with the left or the right hand.

3 Move on to work the HEAD and BRAIN reflex areas on the thumb and fingers with the hook and back-up technique. Search with your fingers for the most sensitive areas. Working these areas can help to relieve tension and pain.

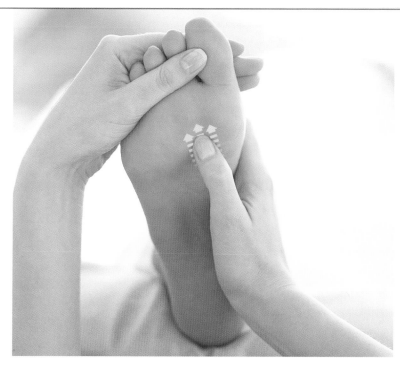

Working the feet

When you are working the feet, remember to carry out the whole sequence on each foot. One foot may be more more tender than the other, which can indicate that more work in that area is needed. If you are prone to headaches, working on your feet regularly may help to prevent them.

1 Begin by thumb-walking through the SOLAR PLEXUS reflex area to relieve tension throughout the body. Make multiple passes.

TYPES OF HEADACHE

Depending on your headache, work the following reflex areas.

MIGRAINE HEADACHE: Thumb-walk along the TAILBONE reflex area on the foot.

MIGRAINE HEADACHE WITH VISION IMPAIRMENT: Walk-down/pull-against through the NECK reflex area on the index finger.

HEADACHE AT TOP OF HEAD: Work the HEAD reflex on the top of big toe.

HEADACHE AT SIDE OF HEAD: Work the HEAD reflex on the side of big toe.

PAIN AT BACK OF HEAD: Thumb-walk the HEAD reflex area on the base of the ball of the big toes.

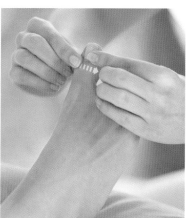

2 Next, hold the toe in place and roll your fingertip over the top of the toe. Repeat on the other foot. Work any sensitive areas you find thoroughly.

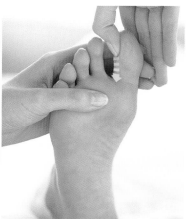

3 To relieve tension in the head and neck, thumb-walk down all sides of the big toe, to the base of the toe. Repeat on the other foot.

BACKACHE & NECK PAIN

Backache and neck pain mean something different for each of us. Start by locating the pain in your body, and then use the foot and hand maps (*see pages 16–23*) to find the reflex areas that correspond to the ache. Remember that tension in muscles and joints frequently contribute to backache and neck pain, so try to work reflex areas that relate to more general areas of tension.

Working the hand

Hand reflexology is convenient for working with backache and neck pain, since you can apply technique discreetly at almost any time.

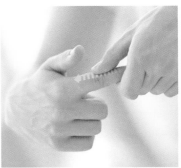

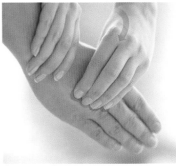

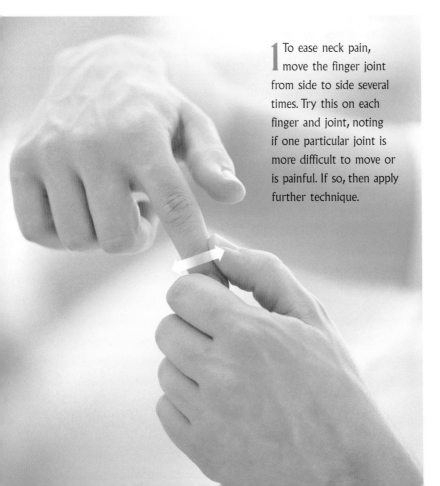

RESEARCH

Several recent studies found that 74–98 per cent of reflexology recipients found the treatment effective for relieving their neck and lower back pain. Self-help reflexology was suggested to continue the benefits.

---

1 To ease neck pain, move the finger joint from side to side several times. Try this on each finger and joint, noting if one particular joint is more difficult to move or is painful. If so, then apply further technique.

2 Now walk-down / pull-against through the NECK reflex area. To increase the stretch in each finger, lower the wrist and press harder with your thumb. Thumb-walk forwards through the area.

3 Apply the palm-mover (*see page 101*) to relax the UPPER and LOWER BACK reflex areas. Press with the fingers while pulling up with the thumb to create counter-movement.

Working the foot

For best results, before you start applying reflexology to the foot, consult the maps (*see pages 16–19*) to pinpoint reflex areas that correspond to the pain. Remember to repeat the sequence on both feet. You may find reflex areas on one foot to be especially sensitive, so target them with more work.

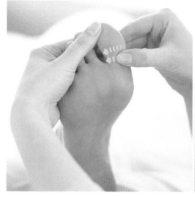

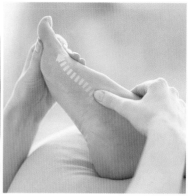

1 Begin by working the NECK reflex area to release tension in the corresponding part of the body. Thumb-walk round the base of the big toe, making several successive passes.

2 Now work from mid-back on the SPINE reflex area to that for the area between the SHOULDER BLADES. Problems in this part of the back can contribute to tension and pain in the neck and upper back.

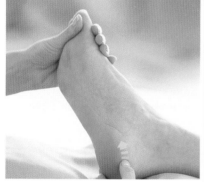

4 Use all four fingers together to finger-walk through the LOWER BACK reflex area. Then, position your hand so the fingertips rest closer to the toes and finger-walk through this part of the foot.

3 Start from the TAILBONE reflex area and thumb-walk through the LUMBAR SPINE reflex area several times. This is a broad area, so cover it from several different angles.

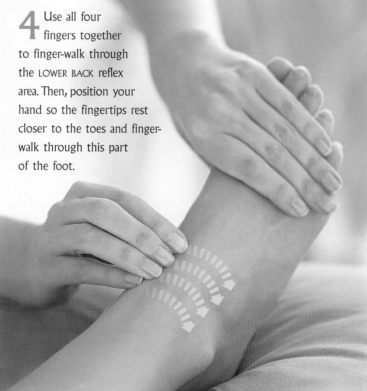

PAIN

In reflexology, pain is addressed by applying direct pressure to the relevant reflex area. First find the area as reflected on the foot or hand. Work that specific reflex area by applying a direct, steady and constant pressure to the reflex area until the pain eases. Working the solar plexus reflex area and applying a full series of desserts also helps to ease general tension levels. However, you should always have any unknown pain diagnosed by your doctor.

WHERE DOES IT HURT?

Begin by noting the location of the pain on your body. Next, find the corresponding reflex areas by looking at the foot and hand maps (see pages 16–23). To orient yourself, remember that the right-hand side of the body is reflected on the right hand and foot, and the left-hand side of the body on the left hand and foot.

Working the hands

Here are suggestions to ease tension, which often contributes to pain, and to relieve pain in the head and chest areas. When you press into the reflex area, avoid digging your thumbnail into the hand.

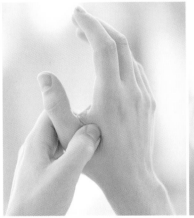

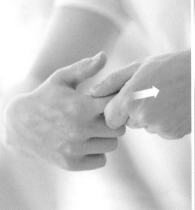

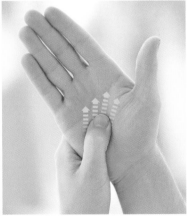

To relieve tension

Rest your thumb and fingertip in the webbing of the hand at the SOLAR PLEXUS reflex area. Press several times.

For pain in the neck or head

To help ease pain, apply direct pressure to the HEAD and NECK reflex areas in the finger or thumb by squeezing the digit between thumb and index finger tips. Hold for 15–30 seconds. Repeat.

For pain in the abdomen or chest

If the pain is in the trunk of the body, work the palm of the hand. Press your thumb into the reflex area that corresponds to the site of the pain. Hold for 15–30 seconds to see if the pain lessens. Reposition your thumb and try applying pressure to the most sensitive area.

Working the feet

First work the solar plexus reflex area (*see below*) to ease tension, and then apply direct pressure to the reflex area that reflects the location of the pain. Here are suggestions for pain in the neck and trunk areas.

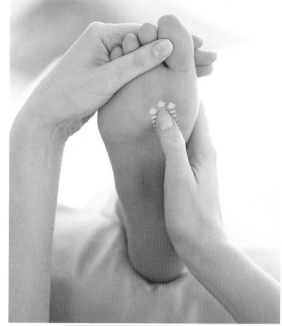

To relieve tension

To relax the foot, thumb-walk through the SOLAR PLEXUS reflex area (*see right*). Go on to apply a full series of desserts (*see pages 68–73*).

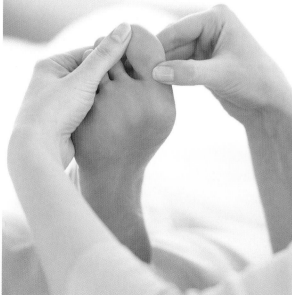

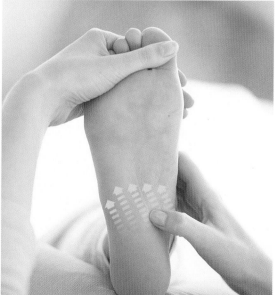

For pain in the neck or head

To help ease pain, apply pressure to the HEAD or NECK reflex sites on the toes (*see pages 16–19*) by pinching the selected area between thumb and fingers. Hold for 15–30 seconds, or until the pain lessens.

For pain in the abdomen or chest

If the pain lies in the trunk of the body, apply technique to the sole of the foot. Place your thumb on the reflex area selected and drop your wrist. Maintain this position. See if pain is lessened with a 15–30 second hold. Reposition your thumb and try again.

ARTHRITIS & RHEUMATISM

Arthritis and rheumatism are characterised by painful inflammation of the joints. These conditions affect the whole body, so work the whole foot or hand. You should work reflex areas corresponding to the kidneys, which help to eliminate waste products from the body, and the adrenal gland reflex areas, since the adrenals help fight inflammation. Working the solar plexus reflex area can relieve tension, a contributory factor in arthritis. (*See also Pain, pages 140–41.*)

RESEARCH

Studies in China, which were reported in 1996, have suggested that reflexology had a beneficial effect on 91–95 per cent of those suffering from arthritis. Self-help reflexology appeared to help maintain these results.

Working the hands

Applying reflexology to the hands for arthritis involves two strategies: one is to work reflex areas associated with the overall condition and the other is to encourage movement of stiff fingers and hands. Remember to work both hands evenly.

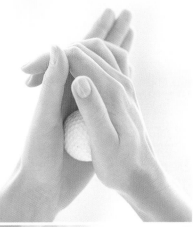

1 Begin by rolling a golf ball over the ADRENAL GLAND reflex area, the general area in the heel of the hand below the thumb.

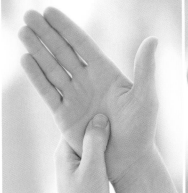

2 Go on to pinch the KIDNEY reflex area with finger and thumb. Hold for several seconds.

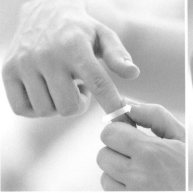

3 Move the finger joints from side to side to mobilise the joints. Work all fingers evenly.

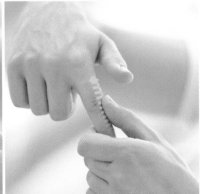

4 To maintain their flexibility, apply the walk-down/pull-against technique to the fingers.

Working the feet

If you are working with someone with arthritis, be gentle, and maintain eye contact to ensure you are working within their comfort zone.

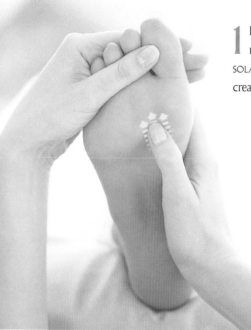

1 Begin by thumb-walking repeatedly through the SOLAR PLEXUS reflex area, which creates a relaxing effect.

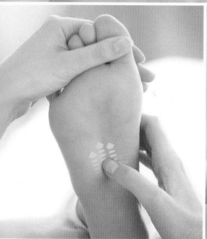

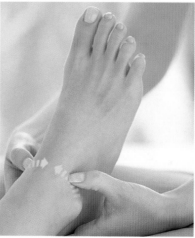

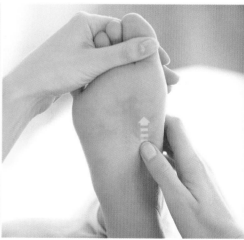

2 Thumb-walk repeatedly along the KIDNEY reflex area. The kidneys can be useful in eliminating waste materials that can gather round the joints.

3 Thumb-walk through the LYMPH GLAND reflex area several times. These glands remove toxins and aid the removal of material stirred up by reflexology work.

4 Move on to work the ADRENAL GLAND reflex area. The adrenals help fight inflammation.

OTHER HEALTH CONCERNS

When using this section, experiment to see what works best. Unless otherwise stated, apply reflexology techniques 3–4 times for several minutes throughout the day, and then repeat on the other foot.

Low energy

Fatigue, particularly in the afternoon, may indicate your blood-sugar levels are low. The pancreas is involved in regulating blood-sugar levels, and working the PANCREAS reflex area as shown 3–4 times a day may help.

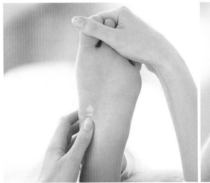

Thumb-walk through the PANCREAS reflex area for several minutes.

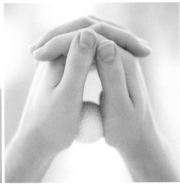

Rest a golf ball as shown. Roll it over the PANCREAS area for 2–3 minutes.

Asthma

An allergic condition, asthma is characterised by wheezing, coughing and difficulty in exhaling. Targeting the ADRENAL GLAND reflex area may help to relieve symptoms because improved production of adrenal gland hormones is believed to help the lungs relax and function better. Using a golf ball on the hands is our favourite technique for asthma.

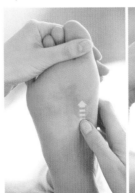

Make several thumb-walking passes through the ADRENAL GLAND reflex area.

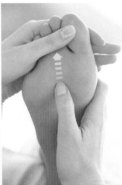

Thumb-walk several times through the LUNG reflex area, and work throughout the ball of the foot.

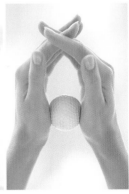

Roll the golf ball, working the ADRENAL GLAND reflex area until symptoms diminish.

Allergies, hay fever & sinus problems

Inflammation is a common symptom of these conditions. Cortisol, a hormone secreted by the adrenal glands, helps reduce levels of the chemical that causes inflammation. To help the adrenal glands function well, work the ADRENAL GLAND reflex areas 3–4 times a day for several minutes.

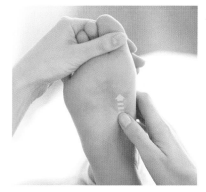

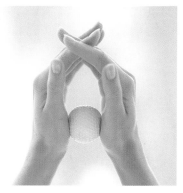

Thumb-walk through the ADRENAL GLAND reflex area (*see above*).

Roll a golf ball round the ADRENAL GLAND reflex area (*see above*).

Bronchitis

This condition is an inflammation of the bronchial (lung) tubes. To help reduce inflammation, target the ADRENAL GLAND reflex areas (*see above*). In addition, working the LUNG reflex areas may also help reduce bronchitis symptoms.

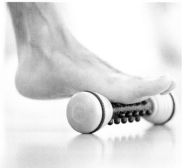

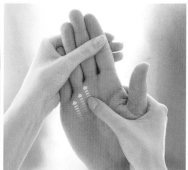

Use a foot roller to work the LUNG reflex area (*see above*). Also work the ADRENAL GLAND reflex area.

Thumb-walk repeatedly over the LUNG reflex area on the hand (*see above*). Then target the ADRENAL GLAND reflex area.

Sore throat & tonsillitis

If you have a sore throat or tonsillitis, you can try applying technique to the NECK reflex area and to the ADRENAL GLAND reflex area to help soothe symptoms and reduce inflammation. If the hand reflex areas are overly sensitive, treat the corresponding area on the foot, and vice versa.

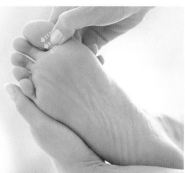

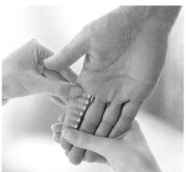

Thumb-walk over the NECK reflex area for several minutes (*see above*). Also work the ADRENAL GLAND reflex area.

Thumb-walk repeatedly through the NECK reflex area (*see above*). Also target the ADRENAL GLAND reflex area.

Tinnitus

This condition causes a ringing, hissing or buzzing noise in the ear. Apply technique on the hand or foot EAR reflex on the same side as the ringing ear and work until the noise subsides. Note how much time is required. Work 3–4 times a day for several minutes as a preventive measure.

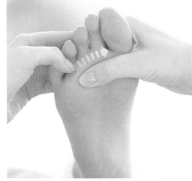

Apply thumb-walking technique to the EAR reflex area.

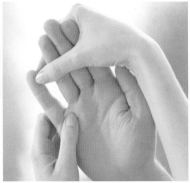

Pinch the EAR reflex area in between the little and ring fingers.

Eye disorders

For eyestrain, you can work the EYE reflex areas until your eyes feel more comfortable. If you have conjunctivitis or some other eye concern, work the eye reflex areas 3–4 times a day for several minutes.

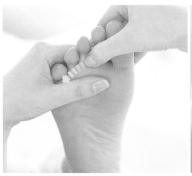

Apply the thumb-walking technique to the EYE reflex area.

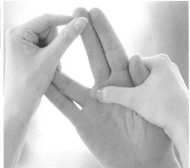

Pinch the EYE reflex area in between the ring and middle fingers.

Skin disorders

For general skin disorders such as acne, working the KIDNEY reflex area may help to aid elimination of toxins that could be contributing to the problem. (*For recovery from painful skin conditions such as burns or shingles see Pain, pages 140–41.*)

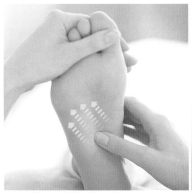

Apply thumb-walking technique to the KIDNEY reflex area 3–4 times throughout the day.

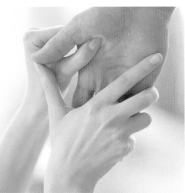

Pinch deep into the webbing in the the KIDNEY reflex area 3–4 times throughout the day.

Heart problems

For heart conditions, 3–4 times a day work the HEART reflex area, the SOLAR PLEXUS area (to aid relaxation) and the BRAIN STEM area (the brain stem regulates some of the heart's activities). If it is inconvenient to work the feet, try working the hands (*see right*).

Thumb-walk through the HEART reflex area (the joint area below the thumb), making repeated passes.

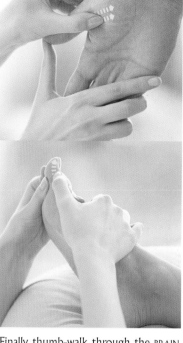

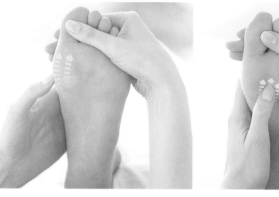

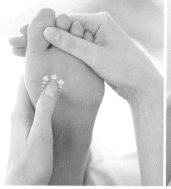

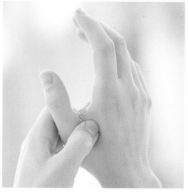

Work the HEART reflex area using the thumb-walking technique. Cover the entire reflex area, which lies below the big toe on the ball of the foot. Make repeated passes.

Now work the SOLAR PLEXUS reflex area, applying several light thumb-walking passes for general relaxation.

Finally thumb-walk through the BRAIN STEM reflex area, making several passes.

High blood pressure

Plenty of relaxation is key for people with high blood pressure. For optimum relaxation, a full foot sequence is ideal. You can also try just working the SOLAR PLEXUS area. Desserts (*see pages 68–73 and 98–101*) have a calming effect.

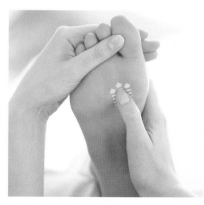

Apply the thumb-walking technique to the SOLAR PLEXUS reflex area for several minutes 3–4 times a day.

Pinch the SOLAR PLEXUS area, in the webbing of the hand. Repeat for several minutes 3–4 times a day.

Fluid retention

The lymphatic system helps distribute fluids round the body. Working the LYMPH GLAND reflex areas in order to help the system work more efficiently may help to reduce fluid retention.

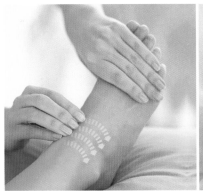

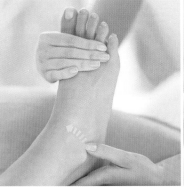

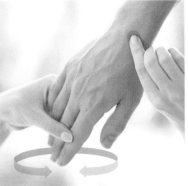

Finger-walk through the LYMPH GLAND and LOWER BACK reflex areas with all four fingers. When you take your fingers away, do you see an indention in the swelling? Go on to work other areas of swelling.

Apply several thumb-walking passes to the LYMPH GLAND reflex area. Pause and note any change in the appearance of swelling. Work through the reflex areas on both ankles, targeting areas of swelling.

Place a finger on the LYMPH GLAND reflex area and rotate on a point by circling the hand being worked several times. Reposition the finger and repeat across the area, before working the other hand.

Stroke

A stroke, which is the result of the brain's blood supply being interrupted (often as the result of a blood vessel rupture) can cause unconsciousness, paralysis and other problems. Apply technique for several minutes 3–4 times a day to the BRAIN reflex area on the opposite side of the body to the side that is paralysed. This targets the reflex area representing the site of the blood vessel rupture.

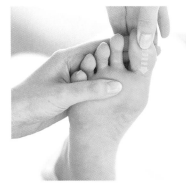

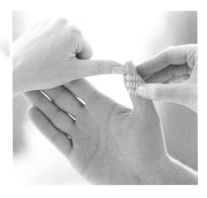

Apply the thumb-walking technique to the BRAIN reflex area on the ball of the toe. Roll the index fingertip over the BRAIN reflex area several times as well.

Thumb-walk throughout the brain reflex area – the ball of the thumb.

Anaemia

This is a disorder in which haemoglobin, the iron-rich protein in the red blood cells, is deficient or abnormal. The spleen reflex area is targeted because this organ controls the quality of red blood cells circulating around the body.

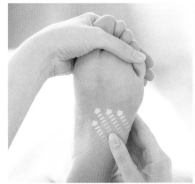

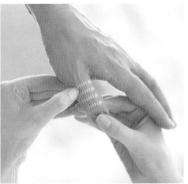

Thumb-walk over the SPLEEN reflex area 3–4 times throughout the day for several minutes.

Thumb-walk through the SPLEEN reflex area 3–4 times throughout the day for several minutes.

Dizziness, fainting & fever

The PITUITARY GLAND reflex area is targeted. For the first two concerns, apply technique until discomfort subsides. For fever, work the area hourly.

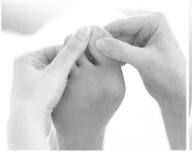

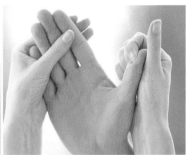

Apply hook and back-up to the PITUITARY GLAND reflex area. If dizziness persists, also pinch the INNER EAR reflex area (*see page 77*).

Apply hook and back-up to the PITUITARY GLAND reflex area. If dizziness persists, also pinch the INNER EAR reflex area (*see page 107*).

Stomach-ache

For stomach-ache apply reflexology work to the STOMACH reflex area until discomfort diminishes. If you are prone to stomach-ache, work this reflex area several times a day as a preventive measure.

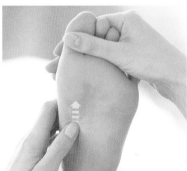

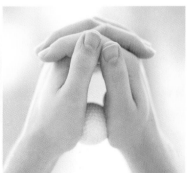

Apply the thumb-walking technique to the STOMACH reflex area.

Use a golf ball to work the STOMACH reflex area on the hands.

Heartburn

A sensation of burning in the oesophagus, heartburn is caused by acid liquid travelling upwards from the stomach. To help bring relief, work the SOLAR PLEXUS area for several minutes because the oesophagus extends through the the solar plexus.

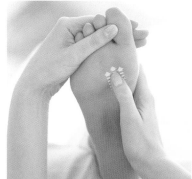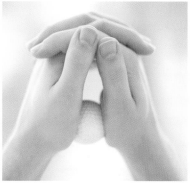

Thumb-walk over the SOLAR PLEXUS reflex area. Apply pressure to any spot that seems sensitive.

Roll the golf ball over the SOLAR PLEXUS reflex area, which includes within it that of the OESOPHAGUS.

Diarrhoea, colitis & diverticulitis

For all these, conditions, apply reflexology technique to the COLON reflex area 3–4 times a day for several minutes.

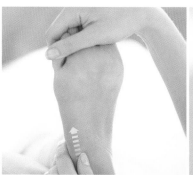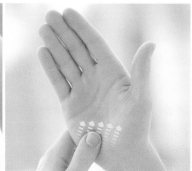

Apply the thumb-walking technique to the COLON area.

Work the COLON reflex area, using the thumb-walking technique.

Haemorrhoids

To use reflexology for haemorrhoids, which are varicose veins of the rectum, you need to work the anus reflex area which lies within the TAILBONE reflex area. Experiment by working this area on both your feet and hands until you find a particularly sensitive spot. Target this with reflexology work.

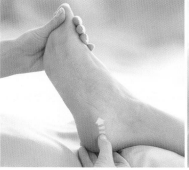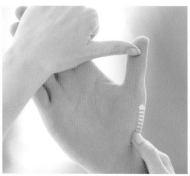

Apply the thumb-walking technique to the TAILBONE reflex area and heel 3–4 times a day for several minutes.

Make repeated thumb-walking passes through the TAILBONE reflex area. Try the other hand as well.

Bladder & kidney infections

For these health concerns, apply reflexology technique to the KIDNEY and BLADDER reflex areas and (to help fight inflammation) to the ADRENAL GLAND reflex area. If the reflex area on the hand is overly sensitive, work the foot instead, and vice versa.

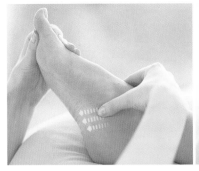

Thumb-walk over the BLADDER reflex area 3–4 times a day. Also apply reflexology technique to the ADRENAL GLAND reflex area (*see page 80*).

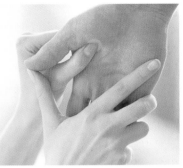

Make several passes over the KIDNEY reflex area. Also apply reflexology technique to the ADRENAL GLAND reflex area (*see page 104*).

Diabetes & hypoglycaemia (low blood sugar)

Insulin, a hormone made by the pancreas, is needed to metabolise sugar in the body. In some forms of diabetes, too little insulin is produced, allowing blood-sugar levels to rise to potentially dangerous levels. For both diabetes and hypoglycaemia, the PANCREAS reflex area is targeted and also the KIDNEY area to help eliminate toxins.

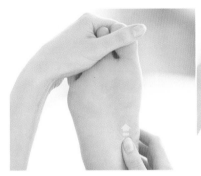

Work the PANCREAS reflex area, making successive thumb-walking passes, particularly on the left foot.

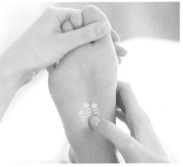

Apply the thumb-walking technique repeatedly to the KIDNEY reflex area. Work both feet evenly.

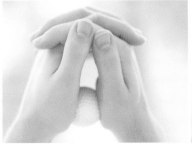

Roll a golf ball over the PANCREAS reflex area several times a day. If the surface of the golf ball is too hard for your hands, use it only briefly.

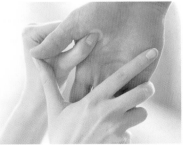

With your finger and thumb pinch the KIDNEY reflex area, repeatedly pressing deep into the webbing of the hand.

> ### CAUTION
> Do not over-work the PANCREAS reflex area – apply pressure only briefly and gently.

Sciatica

If the sciatic nerve is compressed, it can cause pain, known as sciatica, in the buttock and leg. Reflexology technique is applied to the SCIATIC NERVE reflex area. For pain on the left side of the body, work the left hand or foot. For pain on the right side, work the right hand or foot.

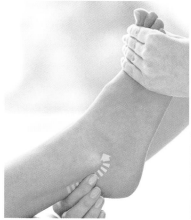

Apply the finger-walking technique to the SCIATIC NERVE reflex area 3–4 times throughout the day.

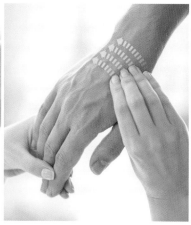

Use all four fingers to finger-walk across the LOWER BACK and SCIATIC NERVE reflex areas.

Menstrual cramps & PMS

Pain and other symptoms are common during or prior to menstrual periods. For PMS, work the UTERUS reflex area on the feet or hands every day throughout the month. For painful periods, work the same area on the hands or the feet 3–4 times a day until the pain subsides.

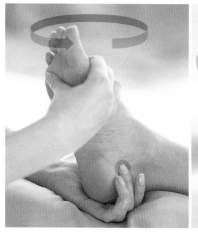

Rest your finger on the UTERUS reflex area, and apply the rotating on a point technique (*see page 66*). Go on to work the other foot.

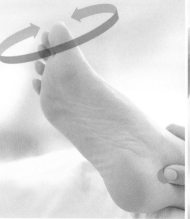

Pressing your thumb into the UTERUS reflex area, turn your ankle in circles, first clockwise and then anti-clockwise. Go on to work the other foot.

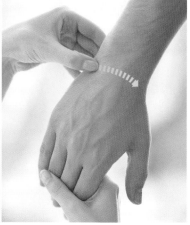

Place your thumb on the OVARY reflex area. Thumb-walk through the area making several passes.

Insomnia

Whether you are unable to get off to sleep or wake too early, reflexology can help treat insomnia. For best results, ask a partner or friend to work on your feet just before bedtime. Follow with a relaxing series of desserts (*see pages 68–73*).

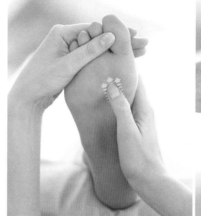

Make successive light thumb-walking passes over the SOLAR PLEXUS area on both feet.

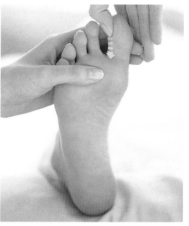

Thumb-walk over the HEAD and BRAIN reflex areas. Also, make several passes over the BRAIN STEM area to encourage relaxation (*see page 85*).

Anxiety & depression

Relaxation is important for these conditions. Work the SOLAR PLEXUS reflex area for relaxation, the PANCREAS reflex area to help stabilise blood-sugar levels and the ADRENAL GLAND reflex area to normalise adrenaline production.

Work the SOLAR PLEXUS reflex area by pinching the webbing of the hand. Repeat several times.

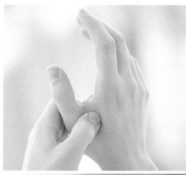

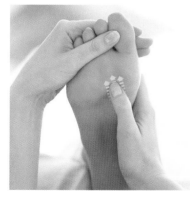

Apply the thumb-walking technique repeatedly to the SOLAR PLEXUS area, using light pressure only.

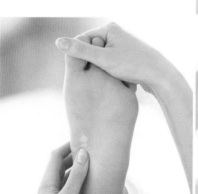

Work the PANCREAS reflex area by using the thumb-walking technique. Make several passes.

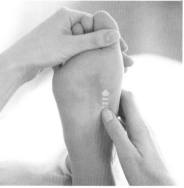

Finally, thumb-walk through the ADRENAL GLAND area several times.

RESOURCES

Finding a practitioner

You may want to hire a reflexology professional instead of, or in addition to, home-application of reflexology techniques. Check your practitioner's credentials for any qualifications and membership of reflexology organisations (*see below*). However, standards have changed over the past decade, so you should ask a prospective practitioner the date and duration of their study, and how much professional experience they have. The best-qualified reflexologists have completed a course of study of 50 hours or more and also have at least a year's experience of practice. It is also worth noting that someone who has expanded into other areas (such as selling products or offering other complementary therapies) may not be as experienced in giving reflexology sessions as a specialist (*see also pages 36–37*).

Contacts

United Kingdom

Association of Reflexologists
27 Old Gloucester Street
London, WCIN 3XX
Phone: 0870 5673320
Email: aor@reflexology.org

British Reflexology Association
Monks Orchard, Whitbourne
Worcester, WR6 5RB
Phone: 01886 821207
Web: www.britreflex.co.uk

International Federation of Reflexologists
78 Edridge Road, Croydon
Surrey, CRO IEF
Phone: 0208 645 9134

International Institute of Reflexology (UK)
255 Turleigh, Bradford-on-Avon
Wiltshire, BA15 2HG
Phone: 01225 865899

Republic of Ireland

Irish Reflexologists' Institute
The Secretary
1 St Anne's Cottages, Gold Links Road
Bettystown, Co. Meath
Phone: 44 28 41 0886777
Email: editor@reflexology.ie

National Register of Reflexologists (Ireland)
The Registrar, Unit 13, Upper Mall
Terryland Retail Park
Headford Road, Galway
Phone: 353 91 568844

Australia

Reflexology Association of Australia
P.O. Box 366, Cammeray
NSW 2062
Phone: 61 02 4721 4752
Fax: 61 02 9631 3287
Web: www.raansw.com.au

International Council of Reflexologists
P.O. Box 1032
Bondi Junction
NSW
Phone: 61 612 9300 9391
Fax: 61 612 9300 9216

New Zealand

The New Zealand Institute of Reflexologists Inc.
253 Mount Albert Road, Mount Roskill
Auckland

New Zealand Reflexology Association
P.O. Box 31 084
Auckland 9
Phone: 64 9 486 1918
Fax: 64 9 489 2916

Websites

www.reflexology-research.com
Kevin and Barbara Kunz's website; offers the basics on reflexology theory and practice, complete with information on developments in reflexology research.

www.foot-reflexologist.com
Kevin and Barbara Kunz offer information and advice for professional reflexologists.

www.myreflexologist.com
Offers interactive information on reflexology products and practice.

www.reflexology.org
Features links to important reflexology websites, as well as a list of worldwide reflexology organisations.

www.iol.ie/~footman/booklst.html
Lists useful reflexology books, videos, and charts and where to purchase them.

www.foot.com
Information on how to take care of your feet.

Further reading

Bayly, Doreen
Reflexology Today
(Inner Traditions Intl Ltd, 1989)

Gillanders, Ann
Reflexology: A Step-by-Step Guide
(Element Books, 1997)

Hall, Nicola
Reflexology: A Way to Better Health
(Newleaf, 2001)

Jora, Jurgen
Foot Reflexology: A Visual Guide for Self-Treatment
(St. Martin's Press, 1991)

Kunz, Kevin and Barbara
My Reflexologist Says Feet Don't Lie
(Reflexology Research Project Press, 2001)

Kunz, Kevin and Barbara
Hand Reflexology Workbook (Revised)
(Reflexology Research Project Press, 1999)

Kunz, Kevin and Barbara
The Complete Guide to Foot Reflexology
(Reflexology Research Project Press, 1993)

Kunz, Kevin and Barbara
Hand and Foot Reflexology: A Self-Help Guide
(Simon & Schuster, 1992)

Advanced reading

Lett, Anne
Reflex Zone Therapy for Healthcare Professionals
(Churchill Livingstone, 2000)

Marquardt, Hanne
Reflex Zone Therapy of the Feet
(Inner Traditions Intl Ltd, 1996)

Eugster, Father Josef
The Rwo Shur Health Method:
A Self Study Book on Foot Reflexology
(Geraldine Co., 1988)

INDEX